# CHOLERA

*The Victorian Plague*

Dedicated to my parents, Dulcie and Lewis Jones,
with love.

# CHOLERA

## *The Victorian Plague*

Amanda J. Thomas

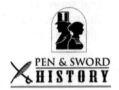

PEN & SWORD
HISTORY

First published in Great Britain in 2015
and republished in this format in 2020 by
PEN AND SWORD HISTORY
*an imprint of*
Pen and Sword Books Ltd
47 Church Street
Barnsley
South Yorkshire S70 2AS

ISBN 978 1 52678 181 9

Printed and bound in England
by CPI Group (UK) Ltd, Croydon, CR0 4YY

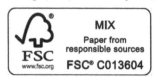

MIX
Paper from
responsible sources
FSC® C013604

Typeset in Times New Roman by CHIC GRAPHICS

Pen & Sword Books Ltd incorporates the imprints of Pen & Sword
Archaeology, Atlas, Aviation, Battleground, Discovery,
Family History,  History, Maritime, Military, Naval, Politics, Railways,
Select, Social History, Transport, True Crime, Claymore Press,
Frontline Books, Leo Cooper, Praetorian Press, Remember When,
Seaforth Publishing and Wharncliffe.

*For a complete list of Pen and Sword titles please contact*
Pen and Sword Books Limited
47 Church Street, Barnsley, South Yorkshire, S70 2AS, England
E-mail: enquiries@pen-and-sword.co.uk
Website: www.pen-and-sword.co.uk

# Contents

**Chapter 9 Cholera Returns:**
The 1866 East End cholera outbreak and the *Princess Alice*

# Acknowledgements

Dr Andrew Ashbee, David Auger, Michael Baker, Alice Barrigan, Heather Burnett, Brenda Clewley, Dr Julie Cliff, Professor Gordon Dougan, Linda Eberst, Ian Ellison, Sam Elvin, Dr Ralph Frerichs, Professor Christopher Hamlin, Laurence Marsteller MD, Professor Roger Pickup, Susan Mary Polden, Helen Rees, Professor David A. Sack, Professor Nicholas Thomson.

I must also acknowledge the experience, help and support of my Editors, Jen Newby and Eloise Hansen at Pen and Sword Books. Thanks also to my family, David, Alexander and Georgina Thomas, who continue to love, support and inspire me.

# Preface

Many years ago I lived in London's Soho, in a sixth-floor flat overlooking Broadwick Street and the John Snow pub. I was not aware at the time that the living room window looked directly on to the site of the water pump said to have caused so many deaths in the 1854 cholera outbreak. Nearby Carnaby Street was not the tourist destination it has since become, and the area had not yet been re-developed or pedestrianised. It is unlikely, but perhaps possible, that some of the pipes through which our drinking water flowed were those investigated by Dr John Snow, in his quest to prove to the scientific world that cholera was a waterborne disease.

Snow did not have all the answers, and today epidemiologists continue his struggle to fully understand the complexity of a disease which still kills thousands every year and is now endemic in many parts of the world. One of the most recent outbreaks began in Haiti in 2010, and since then more than 800,000 people there have been infected with cholera-like diarrhoea, and over 10,000 have died. It is extraordinary that in 2020 almost a billion people worldwide do not have access to safe drinking water, still the most effective way to prevent cholera. Of equal importance is good hygiene, including careful food handling and diligent hand washing, as the recent rapid spread of the coronavirus, COVID-19 has shown. Global warming may also be playing a part, with a rise in coastal and estuarine water temperatures potentially triggering future cholera outbreaks. It may be impossible to ever eradicate infectious diseases, but there is much we can do to prevent their spread.

My own interest in the free-swimming planktonic bacillus known as *Vibrio cholerae* began some time ago, when a family historian asked me why so many of her ancestors had died in London in 1849. 'It must have been an epidemic of some sort,' I replied. This was the starting point for my own fascination with cholera.

Amanda Thomas,
Harpenden, February 2020.

# Introduction

Five hundred years before cholera reached Britain's shores, another epidemic had ravaged the population. As no formal registration of deaths was in place until 1837, we will never know exactly how many perished in the Black Death between 1347 and 1351, but it is estimated that in Europe some 30 to 50 million people died,[1] including around one and a half million in Britain, more than a third of the population. During the same period the plague killed or displaced over half the citizens of London.[2]

Plague epidemics occurred roughly every 20 to 30 years until 1666.[3] In the medieval period, so great was the rate of mortality in the British Isles that the structure of society began to change. The decline in the population meant that the land could no longer be farmed in the same way and in some cases whole villages were abandoned. It is not surprising, therefore, that the plague became an indelible part of the collective memory, fuelling British folklore and creating a deep-rooted fear of epidemic disease.

Recent analysis of the remains of London's fourteenth century plague victims, and research into the *Yersinia pestis* genome, has revealed that the high mortality during this outbreak did not occur simply because the plague bacterium was a particularly virulent strain. Rather the circumstances and a particular combination of factors provided the opportunity for the disease to spread rapidly. Comparisons can be drawn between the pattern of events during the medieval plague and Victorian cholera epidemics, which could potentially explain why cholera devastated nineteenth century Britain.

Plague took hold of a population already weakened by hunger. The Great Famine of 1315 to 1317 began with a wet spring, which hampered the germination of crops, and this pattern continued throughout the summer with torrential rain and flooding. There was a shift in the climate to cooler, wetter weather, and on the Continent the production of crops was seriously affected for around seven years.[6] It has been suggested that the climate change that occurred at this time (and which ushered in the so-called 'Little Ice Age') may have been caused by volcanic activity, possibly from New Zealand's Mount Tarawera, which erupted in about 1314. Cooling temperatures caused crop failure, which in turn led to famine and the compromised health of the general population.

Climate change may have favoured the plague bacteria, but living conditions amongst the general populace also played an important part in its spread. It is now understood that plague was able to disperse so quickly through communities because it had developed into a new type of disease: a pneumonic strain. Had the population of fourteenth century London not been living cheek by jowl in tight-knit, insanitary conditions, the disease might not have taken this turn. However, a combination of all these factors enabled the plague to spread with an unbridled voracity.

In 1722, almost 60 years after the 1665 plague epidemic, Daniel Defoe described the speed with which the disease struck and the fear it instilled within the population:

> 'A certain Citizen who had liv'd safe and untouch'd, till the Month of September, when the Weight of the Distemper lay more in the City than it had done before, was mighty cheerful ... Says another Citizen ... "Do not be too confident ... it is hard to say who is sick and who is well; for we see Men alive, and well to outward Appearance one Hour, and dead the next."
>
> "That is true," says he, "I do not think myself secure, but I do hope I have not been in Company with any Person that there has been any Danger in."
>
> "No!" Says his Neighbour, "was not you at the Bull-head Tavern in Gracechurch Street with Mr. —— the night before last?"
>
> "Yes ... I was, but there was no Body there, that we had any Reason to think dangerous ... Why he is not dead, is he! ... Then I am a dead Man too," and went Home immediately, and sent for a neighbouring Apothecary to give him something preventative, for he had not yet found

*himself ill; but the Apothecary opening his Breast, fetch'd*
*a Sigh, and said no more, but this, "Look up to God;" and*
*the man died in a few Hours.'* [7]

It has been suggested that Defoe's account of the epidemic, *A Journal of the Plague Year*, is based on the diaries of his uncle, Henry Foe.[8] The descriptions of the rapid progression of the disease are reminiscent of the way in which cholera also strikes without warning and kills at speed. Prior to the nineteenth century, outbreaks of pathogenic cholera were rare beyond its ancestral home, the Bay of Bengal and the River Ganges in India. No one knows exactly what caused the disease to spread to the rest of the world in the early years of the nineteenth century, but, once more, the most likely theory is that it was probably a combination of factors, perhaps similar to those which had triggered the mid-fourteenth century plague.

It is possible that irrigation work undertaken in India by the British disrupted, or in some way changed the ecology of the rivers or soil, causing the disease to spread.[9] An additional factor may have been the eruption of Mount Tambora on the Indonesian island of Sumbawa, in April 1815. Graded 7 on the Volcanic Explosivity Index, it was a super-colossal eruption – one of the largest in recorded history. The quantity of matter spewed out from the volcano was considerable, estimated at an ejecta volume of about 160 cubic kilometres; enough to have caused significant disruption to the earth's weather patterns.[10] The eruption may also have affected air and water temperatures in the Bay of Bengal, where cholera is believed to have originated.

The eruption of Mount Tambora coincided with low solar activity, and during the following year summer temperatures in Europe and North America were considerably lower than normal. 1816 was known as the 'Year Without a Summer'. Livestock suffered, harvests were poor, and corn prices rose, at a time when the British economy was also seriously affected by trade restrictions imposed during the 1799 – 1815 Napoleonic Wars. Starvation soon followed for the poorest in society, and caused many to move from rural to urban areas.

Britain's towns and cities started to fill up, and some of the most popular areas to live for working people were around the banks of the estuaries and rivers, where trade of every kind flourished and boats and ships were arriving from overseas at faster speeds than ever before. Such places soon became overcrowded, and workers were crammed into filthy, insanitary tenements. These provided the ideal conditions for cholera, as described in an 1847 edition of *The Times*:

> 'It is now well known that in low, dirty, filthy, overcrowded streets, the attacks of cholera are most frequent, and that the agricultural villages are comparatively free from its ravages. Again, the character of the disease is much less severe in the country than in the crowded lanes and blind courts of a large town ... The same remarks apply both to India and to Europe ... the dirty streets, the badly ventilated houses and workshops, the overcharged graveyards, with their putrid masses a few inches only below the surface in the midst of the living, continually emitting a poisonous gas; the filthy gutters, the badly constructed sewers, the over-flowing cesspools under the houses; the want of air, light, water ... show why death is so busy in the metropolis, and other large towns.'[11]

The social commentator John Glyde was correct when he wrote in 1850 that 'disease is the inseparable associate of sanitary neglect.'[12] Yet, improved sanitary conditions alone were not enough to win the fight against disease, as the Bristol-based physician Dr William Budd realised in his quest to eradicate cholera and typhoid fever. Considered by many to be the founder of epidemiology, Budd was instrumental in bringing about widespread and long-lasting changes in Bristol, which meant that only 29 people died during the 1866 cholera outbreak – one fifteenth of the preceding year's death toll.[13]

Some of the deadliest human diseases are caused by pathogens which can easily adapt and change according to their environment. The pathogens responsible for the plague and cholera, *Yersinia pestis* and *Vibrio cholerae,* are opportunistic and the occurrence of a natural disaster will always make the local population more vulnerable to disease, as evidenced by the 2010 earthquake in Haiti. Since the earthquake over 10,000 have died from cholera and in 2020 it continues to pose a threat to health in the region. There are many indigenous strains of cholera all over the world, living in watery, or aquatic, environments such as rivers and bays. The work of experts, such as Dr Rita Colwell, has shown that the bacterium is highly adaptable and can be present even in waters where there is no faecal contamination. The cholera outbreak in Haiti has ignited a debate, causing scientists to ask whether indigenous cholera can become pathogenic in response to disrupted environmental conditions – also caused by global warming – or whether a cholera epidemic can only be started by the introduction of an external toxic strain.

In the Victorian era there were four major outbreaks of cholera: in 1831-2, 1848-9, 1853-4 and 1866. In the periods between the outbreaks cholera was still prevalent but not so virulent. During the epidemic years did an endemic strain of cholera become pathogenic because of a particular environmental trigger, or was an external toxic strain introduced each time? Within the following chapters, the research supporting both of these opposing views is considered alongside first-hand accounts of the outbreaks, creating new hypotheses and dispelling myths. For example, when Asiatic cholera came to Britain in 1831 it spread rapidly along the coast, canals and rivers. Whilst it has always been acknowledged that the spread of cholera was facilitated by the movement of people from one place to another, the part played by boats, ships and barges transporting goods along the waterways has been underestimated, as has the role of the environment.

Furthermore, in most commentaries, the discovery that cholera is a waterborne disease is more often than not attributed to Dr John Snow. He was correct, but others, such as Dr William Budd, had also come to the same conclusion. In addition, Snow's presumption that outbreaks could be prevented by isolating the single cause (such as the removal of the handle of the contaminated Broad Street water pump) was perhaps too simplistic. Moreover, it is a myth to presume that cholera is caused solely by the drinking of tainted water.

In the late nineteenth century, the improvement of social conditions

CHOLERA

undoubtedly helped prevent the spread of diseases such as cholera. Factors including better sanitation, housing, drainage, waste collection, the building of reservoirs and the relocation of graveyards to rural locations all contributed to the improvement of public health. However, in the fight against cholera, education and awareness, good nutrition and hygiene are just as important as access to a clean water supply. In Budd's words, they are 'of the highest practical importance.'[14]

CHAPTER 1

# An Ancient Disease:
# The history and epidemiology of cholera

Before the discovery of antibiotics in the twentieth century, there was a general acceptance that an illness or infection might prove fatal. Epidemics of diseases such as typhoid fever, tuberculosis, measles, diphtheria and whooping cough were much feared, and despite the discovery of the smallpox vaccine at the end of the eighteenth century, its use was not widespread and many still died from the disease. Yet no single outbreak of any disease was seen in quite the same light as the Black Death of the fourteenth century, which was still vivid in the popular imagination during the nineteenth century.

The prospect of another unknown foreign disease with the ability to ravage the entire population caused considerable unrest in 1820s Britain. Cholera too was seen as a pestilence, breaking out without warning, dispatching its victims painfully and at speed. In addition, just as the plague could be identified by characteristic swellings, or buboes, so cholera left its own deadly mark, rendering sufferers emaciated, with a blue tinge to their skin.

Cholera is ancient in origin and is probably the dehydrating, diarrhoeal disease described in old Chinese and Hindu texts, and by writers such as Hippocrates and Caelius Aurelianus.[1] The pathogenic strain of cholera regarded with most dread has been known by several names. These included spasmodic cholera, Asiatic cholera and cholera morbus, which was the term used in 1629 by the Dutch physician Bontius, to describe the outbreak in Jakarta, Indonesia:

'Besides the diseases above treated of as endemic in this
country, the Cholera Morbus is extremely frequent; in the

15

*Cholera, hot bilious matter, irritating the stomach and intestines, is incessantly, and copiously discharged by the mouth and anus. It is a disorder of the most acute kind, and therefore requires immediate application. The principal cause of it, next to a hot and moist disposition of the air, is an intemperate indulgence of eating fruits; which, as they are generally green, and obnoxious to putrefaction, irritate and oppress the stomach by their superfluous humidity, and produce an æruginous bile ... those who are seized with this disorder generally die, and that so quickly, as in the space of twenty-four hours at most.'*[2]

The English physician Thomas Sydenham also observed the cholera morbus in London during the summer and autumn of 1669. His description of the symptoms sounds very similar to those of the later nineteenth century epidemics:

*'Immoderate vomiting, and a discharge of vitiated humours by stool, with great difficulty and pain ... violent pain and distension of the abdomen, and intestines ... heart-burn, thirst, quick pulse, heat and anxiety, and frequently a small and irregular pulse ... great nausea, and sometimes colliquative [profuse] sweats ... contraction of the limbs ... fainting ... coldness of the extremities, and other like symptoms, which greatly terrify the attendants, and often destroy the patient in twenty four hours.'*[4]

If Sydenham's observations are accurate, then it is possible that a pathogenic type of cholera, perhaps a strain of what would later become known as Asiatic cholera, may have already been present in Britain by the late 1600s. However, as the victims' skin did not turn blue – a characteristic of Asiatic Cholera – it is more likely that Sydenham was describing severe cases of the disease known as English cholera.

Prior to the nineteenth century, outbreaks of pathogenic cholera were rare outside of India. Here outbreaks were more common but they were always localised, and often spread by pilgrims who congregated for waterside ritual gatherings.[5] The first cholera pandemic, or widespread epidemic, began in 1817 and is thought to have started following a gathering of pilgrims at the Hindu festival of Kumbh Mela in Jessore, near Calcutta.

The spread of cholera out of India may have been the result of a combination of circumstances, just as is believed to have been the case with the plague, (as discussed in the Introduction). The eruption of Indonesia's Mount Tambora in April 1815, combined with low solar activity, caused climate cooling and harvest failure. India's population was already weakened by famine and it is possible that cholera initially spread through the consumption of rice cooked in tainted water.

An additional trigger for the outbreak has been proposed by epidemiologist Professor Ralph Frerichs, who suggests that changes to India's irrigation system may have also been a factor in the spread of the disease. From 1801, under British rule, successive and extensive excavations were undertaken in India to free up silted rivers and stimulate agricultural production.[6] The disruption of river sediment, the change of soil composition, and climate changes affecting air and water temperatures could all have played a part in triggering an alteration in the behaviour of *Vibrio cholerae,* the cholera bacteria native to India's water systems which may even have been present within the soil.

The spread of cholera out of India was facilitated by the movement of people, in particular the military, and an increase in trade across both land and sea. By 1820 the first cholera pandemic had spread from Jessore to Nepal, Surat, Bombay and China. It then moved on to Astrakhan near the Caspian Sea, where the severely cold temperatures during the winter of 1823 prevented it from spreading further. Then, in 1826, a second pandemic started in Bengal which took three years to spread to Persia and Afghanistan.

Cholera then followed the caravan routes to Orenburg in the south-eastern corner of European Russia, where there was a pause in its dispersal throughout the winter. Unlike the winter of 1823, temperatures were not low enough to entirely halt further outbreaks.

Cholera reappeared again in the spring of 1830 and began to spread throughout Eastern Europe, Austria, Germany, France, the Americas, East and North Africa, and Britain.[7]

In 1832, writing in the *Medico-Chirurgical Review*, the editor and proprietor, physician Dr James Johnson, described the spread of the disease:

> *'We are rather at a loss for a simile or example to illustrate the journeys of this scourge, which was to go faster than a steam-carriage. It crept, like a skulking hyena, from one dirty lane to another, seizing chiefly on those who were half in the grave already, or who, from terror, were flying before the enemy. It rarely or never attacked those who boldly faced the foe.'*[8]

Britain's extensive influence across the globe during this period meant that the outbreak of any epidemic disease abroad was usually swiftly communicated to the British medical authorities. Cholera was fearfully anticipated, and the rapid pace with which the disease spread caused considerable unease. In November 1831, when cholera had already broken out in the north-east of England, Dr J. Sanders wrote to the President of the Board of Health in London, Sir Henry Halford:

> *'When the disease misnamed Cholera Morbus was confined within our east Indian dominions, it concerned us only as a remote evil – but now that it has traversed Asia, invaded Europe, and advanced to the shores of the Northern Ocean, we awake from our dream of security ... the present epidemic reminds us of one which took a course not dissimilar in the reign of Edward III, anno 1349.'*[9]

The way in which cholera had spread so rapidly, and the devastation it had caused, reminded doctors of the way in which the plague had swept across Europe and into Britain in the fourteenth century. Cholera was an unknown foreign disease which was poorly understood and for which there was no cure; moreover Britain was as vulnerable to cholera as it had been to the plague. The country's working population was, in general, poorly nourished, worn down by a raft of other infectious diseases and living in densely packed housing, with little or no sanitation.

An outbreak of cholera was a deeply worrying prospect, as expressed by Dr W. Macmichael in another letter to Sir Henry Halford, which was published by the *London Quarterly Review*:

> *'This pestilence has, in the short space of fourteen years, desolated the fairest portions of the globe and swept off at least FIFTY MILLIONS of our race. It has mastered every variety of climate, surmounted every natural barrier, and conquered every people ... the cholera like the small pox or plague, takes root in the soil which it once possessed ... Great debility, extinction of the circulation, and sudden cooling of the body are the three striking characteristics of the Indian cholera; these, in the majority of cases, are accompanied by exhausting evacuations of a peculiar character, intense thirst, cold blue clammy skin, suffused filmy half-closed eyes, cramps of the limbs, extending to the muscles of respiration, and by an unimpaired intellect. It is no wonder that the approach of such a pestilence has struck the deepest terror into every community.'* [10]

Fear is perpetuated by ignorance, and in the case of cholera the dearth of knowledge about disease was extreme. In the early years of the nineteenth century, many physicians still went along with the ancient view that disease was caused by an imbalance of humours in the body; others considered diseases to be a type of fever.[11] A choleric humour, historian Christopher Hamlin explains, was 'biliousness ... associated with "a fierce and Wrathful Disposition." That already linked cholera with the tropics, where barbarity reigned and disease was more intense, and with hot and sultry tropical weather that could visit temperate latitudes.'[12]

The *Medico-Chirurgical Review,* reported that some physicians, like Dr George Gregory, thought cholera had been sent by Divine

Providence as a scourge, and it was suggested that if this were the case, then the disease might rid society of 'the drunken, the debauched, and the profligate.'[13] Others, such as the French physician François Gabriel Boisseau, believed cholera was caused by:

> *'The excess at table, abuse of indigestible viands, crustacea, leeks, onions, lettuce, cabbage, pastry, greasy, oily ailments, fruits, cucumbers, melons, farinaceous substances, warm water, wine mixed with milk, old aromatic wine, acrid purgatives and emetics, irritating, acrid, corrosive, vegetable poisons, acids and minerals, the sojourn on board of a vessel at sea; anger and solitude; heat of summer, particularly towards the end of the season; the humidity of autumn at its commencement; the winter season; cold night succeeding hot days; youth and vigour.'* [14]

Doctors were deeply divided in their opinions as to the cause of disease. Some believed infections were *fungoid*, because of fungi found in tainted food and water, others, known as miasmatists, thought they originated in *miasma*, tiny particles spread on the wind in foul smells and odours. Other popular theories were *organic*, caused by a lack of ozone; *electric*, a result of static electricity; and *telluric*, due to poison exhaled by the earth.[15]

In the late 1830s, during the early years of his career, the doctor, statistician, and confirmed miasmatist, Dr William Farr, described the way in which disease worked as *zymosis*, while its epidemic, endemic and contagious forms were *zymotic*, from the Greek word meaning *to ferment*. He did not think that infections worked in exactly the same way as fermentation, but argued that the two processes were similar.[16] Farr believed that non-living zymotic materials were abundant in the urban environment, produced by a chemical process on organic material, and capable of entering the body through the lungs and then infecting the blood, 'the principal site of disease activity.'[17]

In Farr's view, zymotic materials were non-organic but derived from living matter; he theorised that something happened to these particles, particularly in an unhealthy environment, when they were inhaled. He also believed that the characteristics of the zymotic matter changed during an epidemic period, and that miasma could perhaps even generate zymotic material, or non-living organic poisons. Farr identified these most specifically. Smallpox was caused by *varioline*, syphilis by *syphiline*, typhus by *typhine*, and cholera by *cholerine* or *cholrine*.[18]

At the time, the medical world understood that disease was caused by something. The work on inoculation by scientists such as Edward Jenner had demonstrated that disease could be passed from one person to another and was therefore contagious. However, an infection that could be spread in this way was seen as distinct from an epidemic disease, which did not spread out like ripples in a pond and appeared to be confined to certain locations. William Farr's zymotic theory bridged the gap between the old miasmatic idea and bacteriology, which began to be accepted in the 1880s.

Even before the discovery of micro-organisms, the theories of some nineteenth century physicians were remarkably close to the truth. Observers such as Farr could see there was an important relationship between environmental conditions and disease. Cholera was most virulent in the late summer months, particularly during warmer, so-called, 'Indian Summers'. Such conditions favour the life cycle of *Vibrio cholerae*, the bacterium that causes cholera. Doctors treating victims were also aware that something external was being absorbed in some way by the body and subsequently causing the disease.

It is well-known today that drinking contaminated water can cause cholera, but the consumption of shellfish, such as oysters, which inhabit the same polluted estuaries and have a relationship with the cholera bacteria, known as *vibrios*, was also a major cause in the nineteenth century, as were any raw and cooked foods tainted by dirty water. Here cholera bacteria could multiply and be dispersed by flying insects and household pests such as mice. Nevertheless, like all diseases that infect the human gut, cholera is most efficiently spread by the oral-faecal route, and an ignorance of the importance of careful food preparation and good hand hygiene.

Yet, the spread of cholera, and the speed with which it travelled from country to country, was not so much a consequence of the transmission from person to person, but because of the movement of ships along worldwide trade routes. This had been known for some time, as noted by Dr James Johnson in 1832: 'It is curious that Cœlius Aurelianus, who gives the best ancient account of cholera morbus, places sea-voyaging among the causes of that disease.'[19]

The clippers, and later the steamships, which plied the world's trade routes could carry contaminated human waste, either in their bilges or anywhere else where effluent might build up. When vessels docked, cholera would have been discharged straight into the harbour waters, and once the bacterium was established in an estuarine environment, such as the River Wear in Sunderland or the Thames in London, it could then move from one waterside location to another, including rivers and canals.

Cholera is carried within water and can travel considerable distances in tidal locations, but it can also swim independently.[20] In addition, it can be transmitted on to items tainted by those suffering from the disease, such as bedding and clothing, either by re-entering the water system through the washing of such materials, or by these items being discarded into the water. In the nineteenth century, cholera moved swiftly along inland waterways such as rivers and canals, perhaps in the aquatic environment, and also inside the bodies of those unwittingly suffering from the disease, discarding their waste overboard. Whilst cholera was also spread from place to place on foot, by road and later on the new railway system, it is evident from disease maps and contemporary accounts that cholera primarily moved from location to location in the same way in which had crossed oceans: on boats.

The most popular nineteenth century theory for the way in which cholera was transmitted was by miasma. This dominated scientific thought, slowed sanitation reform, and frustrated the work of men like Dr John Snow who were convinced cholera was waterborne. In a world ignorant of the existence of micro-organisms it seemed entirely plausible that foul smells, such as those emanating from filthy water, were the cause of diseases such as cholera.

The lifecycle of the cholera bacterium, (discussed in greater detail below), depends on the presence of aquatic organisms called phytoplankton, which are contained in algal blooms.[21] Blooms can give off unpleasant odours, in addition to a blue mist which often appears to exude from them. These mists became a common sight both before and during cholera outbreaks in Britain and abroad, as described in an 1866 edition of *The Times*:

> '... *a correspondent draws attention to the existence at the present time of this mist at Greenwich ... a similar mist was observed at Varna at the time of the Crimean war and in the West Indies before the outbreak of cholera in 1854 ... It was described by all as "a thin transparent bluish haze hanging over the spot, and not affected by the wind".* '[22]

Some algal blooms, particularly those which are blue-green in colour, contain the harmful toxic phytoplankton, cyanobacteria.[23]

Recent research has shown that Victorian visionaries such as William Farr, whose meticulous observations initially convinced him that something was being transmitted in the air, or *miasma*, may not have been entirely wrong. In the early stages of Britain's cholera outbreaks, those who were first and most seriously affected were people working on the water and living on its edges. For them, infection may have occurred through aerosol transmission, and it is known that cyanobacteria found in algal blooms can be inhaled in this way.[24]

In 2014, British Professor Roger Pickup and his colleagues published their research on the spread of Crohn's disease in Cardiff, South Wales. Crohn's is an inflammatory bowel disease and it had been clear to the researchers for some time that there was a significant association between the epidemiology of Crohn's and the River Taff. Bacteria were also detected in three out of 30 samples taken from domestic showers around Britain. The pathogen was found in the tiny droplets which make up water spray, or aerosols, which were then inhaled into the lungs of humans.[25] The distribution of Crohn's along the Taff resembles the way in which cholera spread in the nineteenth century along rivers and waterways, so might it be possible that the disease could be transmitted in the same way as Crohn's?

Work in the United States by M. Elias Dueker and Gregory D. O'Mullan has also shown that it is possible for vibrios such as the cholera bacterium to be transmitted in water sprays, or aerosols:

> 'Recent studies have provided increasing evidence that the bursting of bubbles at water surfaces introduced by aeration, or other surface disturbances, can transfer viable bacteria to the air. In heavily sewage-polluted waterways these water-originated bacterial aerosols may pose as a health risk to recreators in small boats or residents inhabiting the shoreline ... Molecular analysis ... from isolated bacteria demonstrates that water and air shared a large number of bacterial genera and that the genera present in the near-surface aerosols ... contained water-associated Vibrio and Caulobacter.'[26]

However, cholera does not become pathogenic to humans in the lungs, but in the intestines. Pickup et al's work on Crohn's disease showed that: 'Lung involvement is well described in adults with Crohn's disease ... and the disease in children often begins with a cough ... Initial invasion via the oral route ... may result in chronic inflammation of the intestine.'[27]

Bacteria is able to migrate and move around the body and, if it is contained in secretions such as phlegm, may also be coughed up and swallowed. It would not be impossible for cholera bacteria to be inhaled in a similar way to Crohn's and then find its way to the intestines.

In the mid-nineteenth century, Dr John Snow refuted the miasmatist theory of infection via the lungs in the case of cholera. He had worked extensively with gasses, pioneering the use of chloroform, and during dissections of many cholera victims had observed no evidence of cholera in the lungs. Snow was, however, determined to prove his theory that cholera was waterborne, and the slightest hint that cholera could have been present in the lungs would have destroyed this hypothesis, (as will be discussed further in Chapter 7). Yet,the new research undertaken by Pickup et al shows that vibrios can be suspended in water droplets and that it would not be impossible for cholera bacteria to be inhaled into the lungs and then migrate to the intestines, perhaps just as William Farr had imagined. It is a tantalising idea and whilst it does not in any way prove the miasma theory, it does re-open the debate, as Dr Roger Pickup concludes, 'The miasma theory although fundamentally incorrect had some truths if you substitute the concept of foul air with that of pathogen containing aerosols.'[28]

In recent years scientific research has debunked myths and unravelled many mysteries. The decoding of DNA has enabled researchers to finally understand why the plague swept through London so quickly in the fourteenth century. It was not because of rats moving from house to house, but rather because the plague bacteria had mutated into a pneumonic strain. This, and the work of scientists like Pickup and his colleagues, shows that perhaps we should take more seriously the observations of Victorian commentators, for in their findings lie clues to the true nature of epidemic disease.

Unlike smallpox, cholera has not been eradicated and is a serious threat to health in developing countries. The 2020 COVID-19 and 2014 – 16 Ebola outbreaks show how diseases can rapidly become a worldwide threat; research therefore continues to fully understand cholera and its life cycle. A discussion of the epidemiology of cholera facilitates an understanding of why the disease behaved in the way in which it did during the nineteenth century epidemics, and by bringing together the work of modern scientists, it is possible to explain some of the anomalies, myths and contradictions.

*Vibrio cholerae* (*V. cholerae*) is a member of the *Vibrionaceae* family and is a curved rod-shaped, gram-negative bacterium with a flagellum, or tail, which facilitates its movement.[29] The microorganism was first isolated by the Italian Filippo Pacini in the 1850s, but it was the German Robert Koch who finally confirmed the existence of the pathogen in 1884. *Vibrio cholerae* live in water and are free swimming planktonic bacteria, known as bacilli. They prefer coastal and estuarine environments and attach themselves to other organisms such as plants, filamentous green algae, crustaceans, insects, and the egg masses of flying insects such as midges and gnats.[30] Vibrios prefer a habitat that is rich with algae, phytoplankton, and zooplankton. The exoskeletons which sheath these aquatic micro-organisms are made of chitin, which contains carbon and nitrogen, the essential nutrients for bacteria like *Vibrio cholerae*.[31]

Cholera can also be found inside small marine crustaceans called copepods, which feed on the phytoplankton such as those found in the algal blooms discussed above. Cholera flourishes in warmer waters with lower salinity levels, such as brackish river estuaries, and factors such as rainfall and prolonged sunshine can have an impact on the vibrio's development and even its pathogenicity.

There are approximately 200 serogroups, or types of *Vibrio cholerae* and many of these are of the non-pathogenic type. These strains are still capable, however, of causing 'sporadic, yet significant, gastrointestinal and extraintestinal infections globally'[32] and might account for the outbreaks of less violent English cholera, which were observed by commentators like Sydenham. These non pathogenic strains are known as non-O1 and non-O139 and lack particular genetic elements, proteins, which are the components of cholera toxin (abbreviated as CTX).

*Vibrio cholerae* O1 and O139 are the pathogenic types, which today are known to cause cholera outbreaks. Widespread epidemics are known as pandemics. These can consist of separate waves of disease and prior to 2015 there have been seven cholera pandemics. *Vibrio cholerae* O1 was responsible for pandemics one to six in the nineteenth century and began in 1817, 1826, 1852, 1863, 1881 and 1899. O1 is known as Classical Cholera, whereas the later strain, O139, is known as El Tor, and is responsible for the most recent seventh pandemic, which emerged in 1961 and still continues in 2020.[33]

Work on the genetic signature of cholera, such as the O139 serotype, has shown that the disease can be traced back to a common bacterial ancestor in the Indian delta, where the Ganges and Brahmaputra Rivers converge and discharge into the Bay of Bengal.[34] Serogroups O1 and O139 acquire pathogenicity (CTX) through horizontal gene transfer with bacteriophages, a type of virus, common in the natural environment such as sea water and soil, as explained in recent research:

*'The relationship among local incidence of cholera, prevalence of* V. cholerae *in the aquatic environment and bacteriophage that target O1 and O139 serogroups, was investigated in Dhaka, Bangladesh over a three-year period. The number of cholera patients varied seasonally and coincided with the presence of pathogenic* V. cholerae *strains in water samples that lacked detectable cholera phage. During interepidemic periods, water samples contained cholera phage but no viable* V. cholerae. *These results indicate that seasonal epidemics of cholera inversely correlate with the prevalence of environmental cholera phage. Moreover, cholera phage may play a role in the emergence of new* V. cholerae *pandemic serogroups or clones.'* [35]

In other words, the pathogenicity of cholera depends on its relationship with bacteriophages, not just in the Bay of Bengal but also in rivers such as the Thames in London. Horizontal gene transfer between the two is triggered by certain factors: increased rainfall, higher and prolonged air and water temperatures, salinity, and chlorophyll levels found in photosynthesising phytoplankton.[36] It is important to understand, however, that the phages which share ecosystems with cholera are not the same micro-organisms that cause viral diseases in humans. The coexistence between cholera and bacteriophages explains why in the nineteenth century observers noticed a correlation between the weather and the intensity of cholera outbreaks.

Epidemic cholera has two virulence factors: the toxin (CTX) and the toxin coregulated pilus, known as TCP, which is a receptor for the cholera toxin. The pili are short structures, rather like hairs, on the outside of the rod-shaped cholera cell and are essential to the colonisation of the small intestine by the cholera bacteria and the release of toxins. Two toxins are involved in the main process of infection by cholera and these are called subunits A and B. It is the actions of these toxins and others excreted by the bacterium which allow it to bind to the intestinal wall and eventually cause penetration.

27

The release of an additional enzyme by the bacterium encourages the production of water and electrolytes by the body. The cholera bacteria irritate the intestinal walls and capillaries and erode and kill the cells of the lining. The built up fluid containing cholera bacteria and intestinal cells is released and excreted as diarrhoea.[37]

In the nineteenth century, an anomaly, which hindered research and confirmation that cholera was a waterborne disease, was that infection did not always occur following the drinking of large quantities of tainted water. The work of Professor Bonnie L. Bassler in the United States has shown that the amount of bacteria consumed is indeed important, and it is not necessary to consume large numbers of *Vibrio cholerae* to become infected. This explains why many victims became ill after having simply added a few drops of tainted water to a glass of whiskey, or even because they had not washed their hands after dealing with the evacuations of a cholera patient.

Bassler and her colleagues discovered that in order to release toxin, as explained above, cholera bacteria also have the ability to secrete chemicals which they are able to sense and use as a form of group communication. This is known as quorum sensing:

> 'The bacterial communication phenomenon ... is called quorum sensing ... a process that allows bacteria to communicate using secreted chemical signaling molecules called autoinducers. This process enables a population of bacteria to collectively regulate gene expression and, therefore, behavior. In quorum sensing, bacteria assess their population density by detecting the concentration of a particular autoinducer, which is correlated with cell density. This "census-taking" enables the group to express specific genes only at particular population densities. Quorum sensing is widespread; it occurs in numerous Gram-negative and Gram-positive bacteria. In general, processes controlled by quorum sensing are ones that are unproductive when undertaken by an individual bacterium but become effective when undertaken by the group. For example, quorum sensing controls bioluminescence,*

28

*secretion of virulence factors, sporulation, and conjugation. Thus, quorum sensing is a mechanism that allows bacteria to function as multi-cellular organisms.* [38]

Once cholera has infected a person they will suffer from severe diarrhoea, which has the characteristic cloudy look of water in which rice has been boiled. Cholera evacuations are not made up of digested food but rather particles of intestinal mucus and epithelial cells broken down by the cholera toxin, as described above. Excreted interstitial fluid, comprising chloride, bicarbonate and water, also contains some 108 viable vibrios per millilitre and it is this concentration of bacteria which facilitates the effective spread of cholera. The secretion of cholera toxin in the intestine also inhibits the absorption of water and electrolytes, or salts, into the blood and so rapid dehydration occurs.

Many cholera victims dismiss the initial diarrhoea as it is often painless. Nonetheless, this is swiftly followed by violent, agonising vomiting and it is during this final stage that fluid is almost being pumped out of the body. The pulse rate decreases but there is an increase in pulse volume, or hypotension, and the respiratory rate. Victims suffer terrible thirst, a cessation of urination and sunken, wrinkled skin. Blood plasma and interstitial fluid begin to communicate freely, the blood thickens and circulation is inhibited, depriving the organs of oxygen and giving victims a characteristic blue hue. In many cases, death will be as a result of cardiac arrest.[39]

In 1832, *The Medico-Chirurgical Review* gave this description of the process:

> *'The vomited matter in general consisted of undigested food at first, sometimes partially tinged with yellowish green; of fluid ingesta, also occasionally imbued with greenish coloured matter, and partly of slime and mucous. Often, however, it consisted of undigested food, or of fluid ingesta alone, without being in any wise so imbued. In the retching and vomiting which followed, the fluids taken continued to be rejected with a little greenish coloured matter, with or without slime or mucous. The dejections*

*were always watery; sometimes as if coloured with feculent*
*matter; in general they were either colourless, somewhat*
*like whey or had the appearance of rice-water, barley-*
*water, occasionally somewhat dirty, or with an avanaceous*
*sediment, after being shaken in water.'*[40]

During the cholera epidemics of the nineteenth century, as no one knew the cause of cholera, treatment was experimental. Most medicines were old remedies which had been used for generations, such as beef broth, milk,[41] and brandy (further discussed in the following chapter). However, certain mixtures became more popular as medical practitioners tested their efficacy on cholera victims. One of these was calomel, or mercurous chloride, the toxic compound of which was added to water as a purgative.

The London surgeon, Dr E. Manby, described his recipe as follows:'Calomel 1 grain, ipecacuanha [a dried Brazilian plant root] half a grain, opium one qtr. of a grain. All made into a pill to be taken every three hours till symptoms abated which 'they usually did' in 6 to12 hrs.'[42] Another popular treatment was noted down in 1848 by the physician Dr Archibald Billing: 'Water half a pint, tartar emetic two grains, sulphate of magnesia half an ounce, mixed. This dose is for an adult (15 years up) a table spoon every half hour; for a child of a year and a half or two years, a tea spoonful, for the intermediate years a proportionate dose.'[43]

Many physicians, including Billing, noted that a saline solution, (i.e. water and salt), was particularly effective and today this remedy is still used to rehydrate victims as rapidly as possible. It was described in this way by the World Health Organisation, in 2014: 'Cholera is an easily treatable disease. The prompt administration of oral rehydration salts to replace lost fluids nearly always results in cure. In especially severe cases, intravenous administration of fluids may be required to save the patient's life.'[44]

CHAPTER 2

# Brandy is the Cure:
# The 1831–2 cholera outbreak

*'As soon as vomiting has produced its salutary effect on the circulation, or has failed to produce that effect ... I would propose diffusible stimuli with calomel and opiates, but not in immoderate doses. Brandy and laudanum, as the most readily procured, and the least likely to be loathed, are perhaps the best.'*

This advice was published in 1832 by *The Medico-Chirurgical Review,*[1] yet neither brandy nor laudanum was to prove effective in the fight against cholera; during 1831 and 1832 at least 32,000 Britons were to perish from the disease.[2]

Two years earlier, on 27 October 1830, *The Times* newspaper had published chilling news from the British Ambassador in St Petersburg of the 'rapid and fatal progress' of a deadly strain of cholera in the south-east of Russia.[3] At Astrakhan fatalities had reached around 100 per day and the fear was that cholera would soon spread to Moscow, St Petersburg, Warsaw, and then on to Germany. The Privy Council felt that customs officers should be on high alert when observing vessels arriving from overseas, as it would only be a matter of time before cholera reached Britain.

Cholera was by now the talk of Europe, although some believed that it was perhaps the plague that was devastating 'the territories of the East India Company.'[4] The *London Medical Gazette* noted on 18 June 1831: 'This subject divides attention with the reform bill. No medical man can enter a house without being questioned about it; and the papers, both at home and abroad, teem with the most alarming accounts. In short, there is complete panic.'[5]

The Clerk of the Privy Council despatched Dr Thomas Walker to Russia to investigate, and he concluded that the disease from which so many were dying was indeed the cholera morbus. Walker reported:

> 'In Moscow by far the greater part of the medical men are of the opinion that the disease is not contagious, but produced by some peculiar state of the atmosphere, not cognizable by either our sense or instruments ... In the rest of my journey ... through which all places the disease made its approaches towards St. Petersburg ... the medical men and others [were] convinced that the disease was brought up ... by the boats which came up the Volga ... and other places where the disease had been ... the first attacked with the disease were always boatmen, and it was only afterwards that the disease appeared amongst the townspeople.'[6]

Despite his observations, Walker did not see anything wrong in allowing ships to travel from Russia to Britain and he made no case for quarantining such vessels. He was of the opinion that cholera did not appear to have the ability to remain dormant in humans for longer than 14 days, and for that reason there was no danger in the disease being transmitted. However, Walker admitted that he was not entirely certain about Russian theories on cholera:

> 'I myself am convinced of the contagious nature of the disease, but that the proofs of its transmission from one individual to another are not quite perfect as yet. And believing so, I cannot, of course be without some apprehension that it may also be conveyed by clothes and other articles, which have been in more immediate contact with the sick ... [cholera] must have its own laws as well as the plaque, typhus fever and other contagious or infectious disorders, but these laws we do not sufficiently know.'[7]

A Board of Health had been established in 1805 by the Privy Council, when it was feared yellow fever might spread to Britain, but when an epidemic failed to break out the body was dissolved a year later.[8] Now, in June 1831, concerned by the spread of cholera, the Government recognised a similar need for a central body but it would operate on a consultative basis. Sir Henry Halford was appointed to the new Board of Health, along with six fellows from the Royal College of Physicians and five government officials – a mix of medical and military men. As the epidemic progressed, by October a subcommittee had also been set up to work on preventative regulations, which were to be issued as Orders in Council and also published in the *London Gazette*,[9] to 'monitor cholera, educate the public, and suggest remedies.'[10] The following month the Board was wound up and replaced by the Central Board of Health; Halford was not included, as his views on quarantine were at odds with those of the Privy Council.[11]

Halford was not convinced that cholera could be transmitted via contaminated goods, and believed that specific measures for the quarantine of ships arriving from places like Russia, where cholera was prevalent, were not necessary. In June 1831 he responded to Dr Walker's observations:

> *'We have not evidence before us sufficient to decide whether this disease be communicable by merchandise or not; there are some statements which appear to support the latter opinion, but they are neither numerous nor distinct enough to convince us that this disease [cholera] does not and will not observe the laws which regulate other infectious disorders ... until such information can be obtained ... we think the safety of the community will best be consulted by submitting merchandise to the usual regulations of quarantine; and we can at present make no other distinction of articles than is made by the law established for purpose.'*[12]

Halford's views were tested on 12 July 1831, when a vessel named the *Edward* arrived in the Humber Estuary. Quarantine officials believed the boat to be without suspicion, but then a couple of days later, as reported by the *Hull Advertiser*, a member of the crew began to experience headaches and cramps in the limbs, 'one of the most certain signs of cholera.'[13] A local surgeon, Mr Fielding, was sent to investigate and the authorities' worst fears were confirmed. Thankfully, the patient recovered and the *Edward* was quarantined at Stangate Creek, some distance away, in the Thames Estuary.

With the threat of cholera now closer at hand, three areas were established under the 1825 Quarantine Act for vessels suspected of carrying the disease. Vessels, their crews, pilots and other associated people arriving from areas where cholera was known to be present were also included. The quarantine stations were: Cromarty Bay in the Murray Firth; Milford Haven; and Stangate Creek. Vessels which had recently passed through Russia, the Baltic, the Kattegat Sea or near the Elbe were also to be sent to the nearest quarantine port. These included: Cromarty Bay; the Firth of Tay; the Firth of Forth; White Booth Roads (between Hull and Grimsby); Stangate Creek; the Motherbank near Portsmouth; Plymouth; Falmouth; Milford Haven; Bromborough Pool (Liverpool); and Holy Loch on the Firth of Clyde.[14]

In the same month there were several fatal cases of cholera among female hemp pickers in Port Glasgow. Reports suggested a further case in Greenock, and even that a coachman had contracted the disease at Paddington in London, but the authorities were quick to play down the seriousness of these cases, suggesting that they were merely occurrences of 'ordinary cholera' and not the more lethal cholera morbus, or Asiatic cholera.[15]

Despite such reassurances, news came on 18 August 1831 that cholera had broken out 'in its severest form known in this country' within a garrison at Hull. A soldier had become ill one morning and had died by the end of the same day. Once again fears were played down and an alternative explanation was offered, that the soldier had been drinking for two days and had then slept on open ground. The garrison was sealed off, but there were more cases of 'common cholera' that week in Hull.[16]

By the end of August 1831 cholera had reached Ireland, and the need to find a cure had become increasingly urgent. The medical profession had deduced that the acidity of the victim's stomach was a factor, and so brandy became a recognised treatment for the relief of the disease. J.T. Betts, the French Brandy Distillery of Smithfield, London was already well-known for its production of the spirit, and had formerly advertised the spirit as:

> 'more wholesome in its effects, and its price but 18s per imperial gallon, J.T. Betts and Co. are again induced to solicit public attention to its decided superiority, as attested by three eminent chemists, to whom it has been submitted for analyzation [sic].'[17]

Now, J.T. Betts were swift to promote the medicinal effects of their product in the press:

> 'At a time like the present, when universal alarm prevails, from a fear of being visited by this dreadful scourge ... it behoves every one, not only to observe the strictest precaution in their diet, to avert, if possible, its uncertain and momentary attack, but to be also prepared with the most efficient remedies ... physicians of the first eminence, who have witnessed its ravages, invariably recommend the use of pure brandy as an indispensible requisite; and as they have also discovered from practical results, that in every case of cholera a superabundant accumulation of acid prevail, J.T. Betts and Co. feel it a duty they owe to the public again to point attention to the superior merits of their French distilled brandy.'

Testimonials followed from luminaries such as John Thomas Cooper, Lecturer on Chemistry, Joseph Hume, Chemist to Queen Victoria, and Edward Turner, Professor of Chemistry at the University of London.[18]

By 1837, Betts was advertising 'important reasons for using Betts' Patent Brandy in preference to cognac ... [secondly] because it is used in our Public Hospitals, and recommended ... [for] the most delicate medical cases.'[19] There were also economic reasons for using the cheaper British brandy rather than French cognac, as the manufacture of Betts' Patent Brandy from grain was beneficial to Britain's farmers, who were then struggling in the face of French competition.[20]

Throughout September 1831 the possibility of an epidemic loomed, as cholera edged ever closer to Britain's shores, and by 14 October the disease had taken hold in Hamburg in Germany. Quarantine restrictions remained in place in British ports and further advice from the new Board of Health was given out on handbills and published in the press, advising the population 'for the prevention and cure of this dreadful malady.'[21]

On 20 October 1831, the *London Gazette* published further advice from Sir Henry Halford, with whom the doctors of the day were largely in agreement. The article advised readers of the importance to keep cholera victims warm and confine them to bed. The patient should have their stomach and even their legs wrapped in poultices of equal parts of mustard and linseed. Body heat should be maintained by applying bags of hot salt or bran, and circulation improved by drinking a variety of remedies, including white wine, whey with spice, a teaspoon of sal volatile (a solution of ammonium carbonate in alcohol or ammonia water, commonly used in smelling salts), five to 20 drops of essential oil of peppermint, cloves or the pungent cajeput[22] in water, and, of course, hot brandy in water. Warm broth with spice was also recommended, 'where the stomach will bear it.'[23]

The addition of 20 to 40 drops of laudanum in any of the medicinal drinks listed was noted as desirable in serious cases of cholera. The new Board of Health was clearly mindful that such remedies might not be within the means of ordinary families, and so they issued the following list which contained ingredients costing only a few shillings:

*'Pint of spirits of wine and camphor*
*1 or 2lb mustard and linseed powder*
*2oz sal volatile*
*1oz essential oil of peppermint, cloves or cajeput.'*[24]

The premise of all this advice to householders was to stock up and be prepared for the worst.

A former surgeon in the army medical service, Dr Joseph Brown, wrote on 10 November 1831 to physician Dr James Johnson, the editor and proprietor of the *Medico-Chirurgical Review*, and Dr Alexander Tweedie, a physician at the London Fever Hospital. In his letter, Brown explained how Asiatic cholera had first appeared in Britain, at Sunderland. Brown was later to be considered an authority on the disease:

> *'Early in the month of August, Cholera appeared and speedily became very prevalent. It ranged in all degrees of intensity, from slight bilious attacks, to cases attended with violent spasm, coldness, collapse, almost, (if not complete) arrest of the circulation, white discharges, suppression of urine, and, in short, all the symptoms ascribed by the observers to the Asiatic and Continental diseases. Of these more intense cases, several were fatal, some of them within twelve hours; whilst others narrowly escaped by prompt and skilful medical assistance. Such cases occurred in situations remote from each other; some of them several miles inland – one, for instance, and that a fatal one, a female living in the village of Boldon, five miles in the interior, and remote from the river. Others of the agricultural population suffered in various situations; some certainly near the river, but there were no ships in it at the time, which had come from suspected places.'* [25]

The summer of 1831 had been 'more than usually mild and genial' in Sunderland. Scarlatina was on the rise, as were 'sporadic cases' of 'indigenous cholera.'[26] The local population had noted an unusual increase in the number of young toads in the area,[27] suggesting a change in the normal weather conditions. Then throughout September, October and November there had been severe thunderstorms and an increase in the levels of rainfall.[28]

It was already known that the prolonged heat of the summer and sudden intense rainfall might be portents of a cholera outbreak, and modern research (as discussed in Chapter 1) shows this is indeed the case. Such conditions mimic the Indian climate, and a warm autumn is traditionally known as an 'Indian Summer'. British surgeons who had worked in India were well acquainted with the symptoms of Asiatic cholera and had not been perturbed by previous sporadic outbreaks of disease in Britain, particularly as they did not manifest the same characteristic violence or kill at speed. Above all, no one wanted to cause widespread panic.

It is difficult to ascertain exactly who was the first victim of Asiatic cholera in Britain, though contemporary commentators believed it to have been 12-year-old Isabella Hazard, who died in Sunderland in October 1831. In his 1832 account of the outbreak, Sunderland surgeon Dr William Reid Clanny recounted how he had visited Isabella at her home, a public house in Low Street, Fish Quay. At the time, the area consisted of densely populated, narrow, dirty alleyways. The district was the hub of local commerce and industry and by 1820 Low Street had around 41 public houses.[29]

Isabella fell ill on Monday, 17 October, with characteristic Asiatic cholera symptoms:

> '... *excessive vomiting and purging of a watery fluid, attended with great prostration of strength and unquenchable thirst, eyes sunk in their sockets, features much altered, a deadly coldness over the surface of the body, with spasms of the lower extremities, the skin remarkably blue, so much so that the mother enquired "what made the child so black," as she termed it; pulse imperceptible, tongue moist but chilled, and a total suppression of urine. Was in perfect health when she went to bed, and had attended church twice on that day; she took ill at twelve o'clock at night and died next afternoon.'*[30]

Clanny visited Isabella at 4.00 am and prescribed a warm bath, brandy and hot water, mustard 'cataplasms' to her calves and a solution of ammonium carbonicum and 'aquae menth,' or mint waters. These were to be taken every hour. Clanny repeated the procedures at 7.00 am and visited her again at 11.00 am,[31] before she died at 4.00 pm.

By Sunday, 23 October, 60-year-old keelman William Sproat had also fallen ill. His house near Long Bank was a 'musket shot away'[32] from the house where Isabella Hazard's family lived. At Sproat's, Clanny met Dr James Butler Kell, surgeon to the 82nd Regiment, also known as The Prince of Wales's Volunteers.[33] The regiment had previously been in Mauritius, where Kell had seen cholera, and he recognised the tell-tale symptoms in Sproat. It is tempting to suggest that since they were stationed in Sunderland, that very same regiment may have played a role in bringing cholera to Britain.

According to Clanny, Sproat had been ill with diarrhoea for a week to ten days, and so he may have been infected prior to Isabella Hazard. Only on Wednesday, 19 October had his condition worsened and by the next day he was 'vomiting and purging.'[34] By 22 October Sproat was greatly improved but, contrary to Clanny's advice to consume only 'farinaceous food,'[35] he had eaten toasted cheese for supper. This, combined with the mutton chop he ate the following day, had a dire effect. After Sproat returned to his boat on the river, the stomach cramps began again. By the time Clanny was called the following morning, Sproat's symptoms were almost identical to those of Isabella Hazard, and whilst Clanny continued to visit and prescribe all sorts of remedies – including brandy – William Sproat died on Wednesday, 26 October.

The following day, Clanny and Kell visited Sproat's son, also William. He was to be found in a damp cellar at Fish Quay, suffering with the same symptoms as his father and Isabella Hazard: severe vomiting and diarrhoea. He was admitted to the local infirmary, where he was put into a warm bath and then given brandy, opium and 'hot substances applied to different parts of the body.'[36] His daughter, Margaret, had fallen ill on 26 October and she was admitted to the infirmary a day later. Margaret responded to treatment and, according to Clanny's notes, was administered with wine rather than brandy. Her father died on 31 October and just four hours later Eliza Turnbull, the nurse who had taken Sproat's body to the mortuary, started to vomit. Her demise was rapid and she died the following day.

On Saturday, 12 November 1831, *The Times* published a report from Sunderland giving details of the latest fatalities: four deaths and seven new cases. The article also listed the surnames of some of those known to have died in Sunderland, including the following new names: Mr Ellimore, Mr Stafford, Mrs Wilson, Mrs Wardle and Mrs Nicholson. This naturally leads to the conclusion that any statistics then being compiled certainly did not include all the fatalities, and neither did any list contain deaths prior to 19 October.

In the same report *The Times* described the case of shoemaker Robert Rottenburgh (or Roddenbury) aged 35. The newspaper not only discusses his death, but also describes his post mortem in some detail. Rottenburgh, like many of the other cholera victims, lived by the River Wear, on the northern shore at Monkwearmouth. Clanny noted that he was a temperate man but liable to stomach complaints.[37] The shoemaker's symptoms were violent and his 'purging ... filled several chamber pots.'[38] Before twenty-four hours had elapsed, Rottenburgh was dead, though, as *The Times* pointed out, his 'mental faculties were perfect to the last.'[39]

It is interesting to consider whether this comment was made to assure readers that should they catch cholera they would not lose their minds, or rather whether it was intended to stress that the Sunderland shoemaker had been conscious of his impending demise. It is impossible to judge, but readers most certainly had an appetite for the most unpleasant of details, as the publication of Rottenburgh's post mortem by Thomas Reddish Torbock, MRCS, illustrates:

> *'POST MORTEM EXAMINATION 20 HOURS AFTER DEATH. Skin of the limbs livid, muscles strongly contracted. The cavity of the chest contained no serum; the lungs were much infiltrated with black blood ... the heart and all the large vessels were filled with black blood, which seemed adhesive to the touch, the cavities of the heart looking as if treacle had been poured over them ... The liver appeared healthy; the gall bladder was filled with bile of a deep yellow colour, like syrup of saffron ... The stomach contained some ounces of fluid like gruel,*

*though a little darker, being tinged with brandy, the smell of which was perceptible'*[40]

No interpretation of what was found during the examination was given in the newspaper, nor in Clanny's published notes, which are drawn on here. From a modern perspective it is difficult to see how physicians failed to realise that cholera victims were severely dehydrated or that the digestive system was under attack. What was clear to them, however, was that Sunderland was in the midst of an epidemic, and of the same deadly strain of cholera which had devastated the populations of India and Continental Europe.

Following the post mortems of Rottenburgh and Sproat the younger, a meeting of the local medical board in Sunderland was convened at 1.00 pm on Tuesday, 1 November 1831. At the time of the meeting, Clanny reported that of the five people who had recently died of cholera, four had succumbed at great speed, and the fifth was nearing the point of death. Chairing the meeting, Clanny asked the gentlemen present to raise their hands if they believed 'the continental cholera' was among them'. All raised their hands.[41]

Soon afterwards, another meeting was held at which it was resolved that:

> '... *medical gentlemen, under whose observation cases of cholera have fallen, draw up a full report of them, and place them, by the forenoon of the 2d instant in the hands of Dr. Clanny, to be transmitted by him to the Board of Health in London. This resolution was carried into effect by ... [Dr Clanny], and the town of Sunderland was immediately placed under quarantine.'*[42]

Yet, later in November there were reports that despite the quarantine, life in Sunderland continued as normal, and as the Bishop of Durham complained to the Secretary of the Sunderland Board of Health: 'I have again received complaints that carriers and other public conveyances are suffered to pass unrestricted to other parts of the county.'[43]

Fearful that cholera was already on the march, London braced itself for the worst. The City of London Board of Health believed that even though no cases of cholera had yet been reported, pre-emptive action should be taken. There was some concern that the narrow passageways of the City could harbour disease, and it was decided that the New River Company should open its sluices and a general cleansing of all the ditches and drains should begin, including a hosing down of the alleyways. It was also agreed that, in order to limit the spread of cholera, the poor should no longer be allowed to roam from one parish to another. The Board was also aware that, as cholera was caused by the movement of bad air and odours, the most important measure they could take was to keep the streets clean, particularly in areas inhabited by the poor.

Finally, there would be no restrictions on vessels arriving in London from Sunderland, save an examination of the crew by a team of specially appointed doctors. The Board could not see the point of restricting movement by water when movement by land had no such limitations. Of greater concern, it would seem, was the financial impact of any restriction on trade.

To ensure that these measures would succeed, the Board printed 20,000 leaflets to be circulated around the City. The leaflets contained advice on cleanliness, ventilation, warm clothing, a good plain diet, abstinence from alcohol, and exercise. It concluded: 'Finally, to preserve a cheerfulness of disposition, a freedom from abject fears, and a full reliance that such measures will be taken by the Government and the local authorities as are best calculated, with Divine assistance, to meet the exigencies of the occasion.'[44]

Much of this advice was sensible, though perhaps difficult for the poor to follow, not just because of varying degrees of literacy at the time,[45] but also because of financial constraints, and their inability to improve rented dwellings. What was clear was that the Board of Health was aware that when cholera struck the hardest hit would be the working poor living in crowded, dirty, insanitary conditions. Yet they could not have known that, by not addressing the cleanliness of the water supply, once cholera arrived in a big city, the whole population would be vulnerable. Worst of all, as the authorities had failed to restrict movement out of Sunderland, the entire country was now at risk.

In Sunderland, the local medical establishment was doing its best to play down reports that Asiatic cholera had started to spread through the city, and were describing outbreaks of the disease as 'aggravated cases of English cholera.'[46] At a meeting of medical professionals, ship owners, merchants and other prominent citizens held in Sunderland on 11 November 1831, there were numerous protests about the unfairness of the quarantine restrictions in place and claims were made that the coal trade was being affected. As a result, the following resolution was taken at the meeting to protect trade:

> *'That a disease possessing every symptom of epidemic cholera is now existing in the town; that it has never appeared on board of ship; that there is not the slightest ground for imagining it has been imported, nor that it has extended itself by contagion ... That it appears to have arisen from atmospherical distemperature acting in most cases upon persons weakened by want of wholesome food and clothing, by bad air, intemperance, or previous disease, and that the interruption of the commerce of the port seems to offer the most probable means of extending the disease, by depriving the industrious poor of their bread, and thus placing their families in the depths of misery and distress.'*[47]

Observers travelled to Sunderland to give their opinions and within days it had been labelled 'The City of the Plague.'[48] Some believed cholera may have already reached Edinburgh, but they were reassured by the fact that careful nursing and the administration of brandy and other treatments had proved effective. *The Times* reported the case of a 17-year-old servant girl suffering from cholera, who had been successfully treated in Edinburgh by an unnamed naval surgeon. A wine glass of brandy and water had been administered, followed by 30 drops of laudanum, 'which she swallowed greedily,' then hot water to the feet and body, a pint of hot gruel and a tablespoon of salt. A fire was lit to keep the girl warm and finally she took five grains of calomel.[49]

There had also been a couple of cases in Gosport, Hampshire, of two seamen on board the naval vessel HMS *Revenge*, but both had recovered.[50] Cholera had most definitely spread and reports of the situation from Newcastle at the beginning of November 1831 were printed in regional newspapers across Britain. In particular, the case of 33-year-old Oswald Reay, an engine man at Mr Crowhall's ropery in Newcastle, was soon well-known and caused considerable concern. The authorities tried to play it down, but Reay's symptoms sounded all too familiar. Moreover, he had died at the end of October, not long after the first victims in Sunderland.

Reay had lived in the riverside area of Sandgate in Newcastle and he first started showing symptoms at around 11.00 pm on the night of Wednesday, 25 October; just over 29 hours later, he was dead. The papers played up the idea that he had died because he had 'refused brandy'; that this was an isolated case; and that he had suffered from such maladies before. Nevertheless, by the beginning of December, as fresh cases began to appear in Newcastle, it was clear that the disease had spread, although it is also probable new cases were arriving via ships travelling from the continent.

The Central Board of Health divided communities into districts and set up local boards on which sat clergymen, medical men and householders. Inspectors were to be appointed to visit the sub-districts daily and produce reports to be acted on. The inspectors were to look at the 'primary elements of public health ... the food of the poor, clothing, bedding, ventilation, space, cleanliness, outlets for domestic filth, habits of temperance, prevention of panic.'[51]

Physicians arrived in Sunderland from London, Edinburgh, Liverpool, Manchester, Birmingham, Leeds, and even France, all curious to learn and to 'observe the character of the pestilence.'[52] Like Kell, Clanny's colleague, many of these surgeons had worked in India and could recognise cholera symptoms. The danger, however, of allowing such individuals access to the sick in Sunderland and Newcastle, was that they too might spread the disease elsewhere on their departure.

There is no doubt that the cases of cholera in Sunderland varied depending on the underlying health of the individual, and the strain of cholera ingested. By the middle of November, the weather had turned colder and reports stated that cases, though abundant, were less severe. However, there were reports that mortality statistics had been suppressed and, moreover, the medical community continued to deny that Asiatic cholera had taken a grip. *The Times* reported that rumours were rife in 'various part of England ... that the people of Sunderland conceal the cases of cholera.'[53] Mistrust in Sunderland also intensified, and the poor refused to attend the cholera hospitals set up by the Board of Health, believing that the dead were being used for dissection and anatomical experimentation.

At the beginning of December 1831, an 'extraordinary fall of rain' was reported in Wakefield, West Yorkshire: 'The quantity of rain ... was so great that the surrounding country was quite overflowed ... about three miles from Wakefield, the water flowed over a wall four feet high; and on the high road near Milne-bridge, it reached half way up the horses legs.'[54]

Such reports indicate that the weather in the north of England was mild in the final month of 1831. As discussed in Chapter 1, these warmer temperatures together with the flooding would have favoured the proliferation of cholera. On 22 December 1831 the Central Board of Health published the available statistics for cases of confirmed Asiatic cholera, revealing that in Sunderland there had been exactly 500 cases to date, with 186 fatalities; 14 new cases had recently been reported. Newcastle had seen 123 cases and 48 deaths, with 11 new cases; North Shields and Tynemouth had experienced seven cases, with five deaths and one new case; at Houghton-le-Spring there had been eight cases, three deaths and no new cases; and from Seghill colliery one new case was noted.[55] These did not include milder bouts of the disease and the surgeons compiling the data did not submit them as speedily as they were supposed to. As a result, it was impossible to map the progress of the disease with any great accuracy.[56]

Reports had also been made a few days earlier of a vessel carrying coal between Newcastle and Aberdeen having requested permission at North Berwick to bury a member of crew who had died of cholera, on a nearby island. Meanwhile, the *Manchester Guardian* warned that cholera had arrived in Lancaster and a coachman and his wife had died.[57] Whether or not such reports of a resurgence of the disease were accurate, cholera, and the fear of it, were spreading. *The Times* coined the phrase 'the travelling cholera,'[58] citing the case on 5 December 1831 of a woman with cholera who had journeyed around seven miles from Sunderland to the village of Houghton:

> '*She was taken severely ill soon after her arrival and died at 5 o'clock today. Oh, what a frightful disease it is! ... Was there ever before such an apparent absurdity as that which allows the inhabitants of Sunderland to travel freely throughout England on the land side with the seeds of this torturing malady ripening in their constitutions, while the intercourse by sea is shackled with quarantine restrictions to the manifest loss or ruin of the shipping interests?* '[59]

A portion of blame for the spread of the disease was commonly attributed to Irish immigrants, as described in a letter published in the *Manchester Guardian* in December 1831:

> '*By means of Irish vagrants from Sunderland, the cholera has been twice brought amongst us. The first suspicious case occurred at a lodging-house in the Half Moon Bank. A man called Mallan, a rambling Irish cobbler, had attended his father at Sunderland, who died of cholera, had assisted in laying out the body, and attending to the last offices; concluding in the Irish fashion by a regular row, getting drunk, and lying great part of the night in the street. This man, coming to Shields immediately afterwards, took ill, and in a short time fell a victim to his folly.*'[60]

This sentiment was repeated in subsequent outbreaks, and particularly in London during the 1848-9 epidemic. Many migrants from the countryside, including the Irish – already blighted by the potato famine raging at home – aided the spread of disease, in part thanks to their habit of keeping pigs in their houses. In Lambeth, local surgeon, John Sewell made the following observations in 1848 whilst conducting his inspection of the area for the District Sanitary Report:

*'The houses in these streets are occupied by the poorest class of society, in most cases by one family in each room. This was particularly instanced in Frances Street which is occupied chiefly by Irish families. In the house no. 28 in that street there are seven rooms, occupied by seven families amounting to no less than 13 adults and 24 children and the Subcommittee were informed that all the houses in that street are similarly tenanted. The cesspools are generally very full and the drainage bad in this district — the privies in many instances full or nearly so and producing always a stench which in wet and sultry weather is almost insupportable and very injurious to the health and comfort of the poor inhabitants. The Subcommittee find that many of the inhabitants of this District keep pigs producing very great nuisance. A man in Gloucester Street has 10 pigs in his cellar and on opening the front door the stench was dreadful, the neighbours generally who do not keep pigs complain of the nuisance of those who do.'*[61]

In 1831 in the North East the poorest in society suffered the greatest loss of life from cholera. Whilst Christmas might have brought a brief period of happiness, the drunkenness in which the population appeared to indulge, either in celebration or to forget the horrors of the pestilence, only served to worsen the situation, as a correspondent to *The Times* protested in January 1832:

*' ... the new disease may be a modern visitation upon drunkenness ... what land ever possessed our religious and civil advantages, and yet so extensively abused the bounty of God in providing corn for human subsistence, by employing so much of it as the great artificial stimulus [i.e. alcohol] of almost all the crimes we witness? In a single distillery at the east of London 45 chaldrons [sic] of coals*

*are burned every 24 hours, while one fire alone consumes*
*5 chaldrons nightly!"*[62]

Not everyone drank alcohol, but in 1849, a general practitioner writing to *The Times* noted that: 'a very large number of persons who have never been accustomed to the use of alcoholic drinks, are now daily resorting to the frequent and immoderate use of brandy and other spirits, with the view, they say, of "keeping out the cholera".'[63] The prescribed use of brandy was not only encouraging those who did not drink to start, but alcohol also created a more conducive environment for cholera within the human digestive system, as it inhibits the production of gastric acid.

Cholera struck suddenly at Gateshead on Christmas Eve. A 'private letter' sent from Newcastle a couple of days later, and published in *The Times* on 30 December 1831, described the situation:

> *'From 1 o'clock on Sunday (Christmas-day) to 10 o'clock*
> *this day (45 hours), 119 persons have been seized, and 52*
> *have died. This is a greater number than the official report*
> *which you will see in the paper, but it is nevertheless*
> *correct. The difference arises from two surgeons not*
> *having made their returns in time. The persons attacked*
> *are all of the poor and needy grade, and possibly many*
> *may have been particularly disposed by the excesses of*
> *Christmas eve,* [sic] *as a gentleman who lives in*
> *Gateshead says he never saw so many drunken people as*
> *on Sunday last; but many very sober respectable persons*
> *(although in the lower order) have suffered.'*[64]

*The Times'* own correspondent in Newcastle played down the number of deaths at the start of the outbreak stating that by 26 December there had been 39 cases and only nine deaths. However, he went on to concede that the situation in Gateshead had most certainly become more grave by the following day, 27 December, as there was already an 'alarming total of 99 cases, 42 deaths and 8 recoveries, out of a population of about 12,000.'[65]

On New Year's Eve, the *Manchester Guardian* carried a story about the sudden outbreak of cholera in Gateshead and re-published a letter from the *London Courier*, in which the correspondent debated whether the direction of the wind had been the cause:

> *'It is difficult to assign any probable reason for this sudden and frightful development of the disorder. Gateshead had been clear of it for seventeen or eighteen days longer than Newcastle, during which time the winds prevailed from the southward. On Saturday the wind shifted to the north – blowing direct from Newcastle to Gateshead; and on Sunday the disease was found raging in every quarter of the town, though attacking scarcely any but the poorer classes of the people. Though the disease is clearly epidemical, there can be no doubt whatever of its being also contagious, and a prevailing idea is that the danger of infection is infinitely increased by coming within the sphere of the effluvia of the dead.'* [66]

The parish of Gateshead struggled to cope with the onslaught of the disease, hindered by inadequate numbers of physicians and supplies. There were not even enough coffins to bury the dead and burials were being performed at such a rate that a new graveyard had to be opened to deal with the increasing death toll. On 27 December, 17 were buried and in addition:

> *'A long trench, capable of holding 12 coffins, two abreast, had been dug, and while the clergyman was reading the service this evening over the first two occupants, four other corpses arrived. Six coffins were deposited in the trench before six minutes had expired. One coffin had a rather remarkable appearance – it was much deeper than the others, and upon inquiry among the friends of the deceased ... they stated that the patient had been doubled up by the cramps, and they had been unable to make him straight.'* [67]

Whilst port towns like Gateshead were susceptible to cholera being introduced from abroad, smaller coastal towns were just as vulnerable and facilitated the spread of the disease. In the 1830s, before the advent of the railways, travel by sea was in most cases faster and easier and short-distance passenger travel by boat was popular. When the Bristol physician Dr William Budd was a student at Edinburgh University, the final leg of his journey from his home in North Tawton, Devon was by sea, from London to Leith on a fishing smack.[68] Laden with cargo and passengers, these vessels and others plied their way up and down Britain's coast. During this period, ships, boats and barges were the only means of transporting large quantities of raw materials and manufactured goods. Their bilges and holds also became repositories for cholera and when the disease arrived in Sunderland it was soon exported to the rest of Britain, along with coal, iron, steel, lead, salt, soda, lime, silver, glass and pottery.[69]

Coal from Sunderland was sent to every part of Britain and cholera may have been spread through the practice of dampening the fuel with potentially contaminated water, to keep the dust down during transportation.[70] Cholera may also have been transmitted on other raw materials which could have come in contact with tainted water, such as clay and sand. Effluent thrown over the sides of vessels would, in turn, have released cholera into the coastal waters, estuaries, rivers and canals, contaminating not just the water but also shellfish, such as oysters.

Following the outbreak in Gateshead, as 1832 dawned three cases were recorded in Haddington near Edinburgh, and by 12 January cholera was reported to have arrived as far south as Stowlangtoft, Suffolk. From Sunderland it spread north to Haddington along the east coast, by ship and boat. From Haddington it progressed to Tranent, Prestonpans, Musselburgh, North Berwick, Leith, and Edinburgh, then on to Newbigging, Alloa, Perth, Stirling and Cupar.

Whilst Suffolk may have already been affected, contemporary newspaper reports show that in the early months of 1832 as cholera spread north it also made its way, step by step, in a southerly direction down the east coast. By April it had reached Goole and Hull, where it may have also been imported within contaminated rags from hospitals in Russia, Prussia, Northern Germany and the Baltic, where cholera was already prevalent.[71] Rags, along with raw human sewage, were used as fertiliser on farms and in this way cholera could also have been spread by the eating of raw fruit and vegetables grown close to the ground, such as strawberries, lettuce and radishes.

The washing of bedding and clothing soaked by the vomit and excreta of cholera victims also released considerable numbers of cholera bacteria into the environment. During this first major outbreak in Britain, cholera outbreaks were initially clustered around waterside communities, where contaminated water found its way easily into food and drink, on to the feet of animals and insects, and, perhaps most crucial of all, the hands of those did not wash their hands before eating. In Sunderland the odds were stacked high that cholera would spread easily amongst the waterside population. Statistics from 1831 show that out of a total population of 9,035 males, 1,586 were employed as seamen, 1,145 as labourers, with a further 1,661 engaged in 'retail trade and handicraft.' [72] A large proportion, therefore, were working on or near the water (where they might also have been susceptible to aerosol infection), and in jobs where their hands were likely to be coming in contact with contaminated water and goods. Good hand hygiene would not have been easy in this environment, nor necessarily considered a priority, and this would have facilitated cholera infection.

Once cholera had arrived in Hull and Goole, it progressed inland along the River Humber to Leeds, via the Ouse to York and Cawood, through the Don to Doncaster, and along the Calder to Wakefield. After Edinburgh, cholera struck in Stirling and Grangemouth and along the busy Forth and Clyde Canal, which was used to transport coal, ironstone, textiles, and even whiskey. Cholera erupted in Kirkintilloch, Glasgow, Paisley, Killwinning, Baillieston, Falkirk, Pollockshaws, Dumbarton, and then found its way across Wemyss Bay to Rothesay. The Forth and Clyde branched into the Monkland Canal which had been completed in the late 1700s to transport coal and iron to and from Coatbridge and the Calder ironworks.

In Coatbridge cholera persisted, as a result of over-population and a lack of a proper water supply:

*'... as the population increased they suffered severely from the want of a proper supply of water. Their principal dependence for this essential element to cleanliness and health existed in the precarious supplies from a few wells in the neighbourhood, several of which during the drought of summer failed in their supplies. There were two or three wells, however, where the supply was filtered into them from the Monkland Canal, and at such seasons of scarcity the people flocked to these from all quarters ... Water in those days, such as could be used by human beings, was often at a premium, and during the few days annually when the canal was run out (which is invariably in the summer) to work repairs on the embankments, etc., there prevailed a famine for water, and the inhabitants were compelled to extremes, and use the dirty, muddy stuff left in the pools at the bottom of the canal, which was enough to bring disease and pestilence into the town.'* [73]

Britain's factories and the network of canals linking them played a key role in the spread of cholera. By the end of May 1832, cholera had reached Yorkshire. Silver and lead were exported from the Dales to Newcastle and Stockton and then all over the world.[74] Cholera spread along the Leeds and Liverpool Canal, the Trent and Mersey Canal (also known as the Grand Trunk), which transported flint from East Anglia and clay from Devon and Cornwall, and on to Manchester via the Bridgewater Canal, Britain's oldest canal which had opened in 1761 to transport coal.[75]

Newcastle's glass-making industry also played a part in the epidemic. Manufactured in the city since at least the 1600s, thanks to a ready supply of coal from Tyneside, glass was packed into crates and transported in the holds of coal ships destined for London. Sand was shipped in from King's Lynn in Norfolk, while fire clay for melting glass came from Stourbridge in the Black Country – another major producer of glass. Clay was transported along the waterways to Bristol, where it was transferred to ships en route to London and, once there, loaded on board the coal ships returning to Newcastle.[76]

The canals were also a highway for emigrants en route to Bristol and Liverpool. At the Mersey port the epidemic killed 1,523 and spread to ships crossing the Atlantic. Outbreaks were subsequently triggered in Quebec and also in New York, where by the middle of August 1832 the death rate was around 80 to 100 a day.[77]

In places like York, local boards of health had not been given sufficient powers to clean up the dirtiest areas of the city, as 'nuisances' were deemed to be the responsibility of the Improvement Commissioners – but only once cholera had already broken out.[78] Until this point any major improvement work was the responsibility of the Commission of Sewers, which was funded by the general poor rate. However, in February 1832 the Cholera Prevention Act finally gave the York Board of Health the power to force local vestries to make improvements, which they were allowed to finance from local poor rate funds. It was too late for them to take any useful preventative measures, as cholera arrived in York in June 1832 and spread rapidly within the water supply drawn by the York Waterworks Company from the River Ouse, which was also the main drain and sewer for the city. York was not a factory town, but home to many small businesses, including glass manufacture, and a distribution hub for the surrounding agricultural land.[79] Once cholera had broken out in the city, there would be little to stop it spreading into the surrounding countryside and beyond.

York's first official cholera victim was waterman Thomas Hughes, aged 21, who lived at Beedham's Court, in a notorious area also known as 'Hagworm's Nest', on the banks of the Ouse off Skeldergate. According to the *York Herald*: 'There were several families residing there for whose use there was only one privy, and at the end of the court was the most offensive dunghill.'[80] Hughes may have contracted cholera in Selby or Hull, as he was employed on the ferry operating between there and York.[81] He recovered, but cholera went on to kill several of his neighbours: John Graves, a sawyer who lived in the same yard; Elizabeth Ward, described as a poor tramp; Mr Barrett, the landlord of Hughes' reputed local pub, the Anchor; Elizabeth Grant of Water Lane; Mr Dobson, a respectable citizen who lived near Skeldergate Postern; and Mary Welbank a poor woman of Nunnery Lane.[82]

Even before cholera had arrived in York there had been much discussion and argument over the burial of the growing city's dead. Traditionally parishioners had a right to be interred in their local graveyard, but in York these were already nearly full. Moreover, there was considerable worry amongst parishioners as to whether their local churches were even safe to enter once the funeral of a cholera victim had been conducted. The problem was resolved with the allocation of a piece of land by the City Corporation in Thief Lane (now close to York's railway station) situated without the city walls. York's problems were also not enhanced by a general lack of sympathy for the poor, who were viewed by more prosperous citizens as filthy and intemperate.

It was seen as inevitable that the poor would be struck down by cholera and local newspaper reports, particularly in the *Yorkshire Gazette*, were uncharitable:

> *'The disease is confined entirely to those parts of the city which a stranger is least likely to resort to; and it is quite evident, that although under certain cases, and in certain habits of the body, the disorder is infectious ... it is not infectious in all cases, as none of the medical men have been affected; nor have any of those individuals who have been employed to convey the patients to and from the hospital, to attend them to the grave, &c. It appears to us that there must be a pre-disposition in the patient to receive the cholera; and that pre-disposition seems occasioned by want of cleanliness, habits of intemperance, and low living, the consequence of poverty and distress.'* [83]

However, during the second week of the outbreak, more affluent members of the community began to suffer. A shift in the tone of the newspaper reports came with the death of Ruth Bellerby (née Hindson). She was the wife of a printer named Edward Bellerby who oversaw the publication of the *Yorkshire Gazette* and whose brother, Henry, was the paper's editor and proprietor. Ruth, along with many others, was laid to rest in the new cholera burial ground in Thief Lane. In the end the outbreak in York killed 185 citizens. [84]

Many once isolated towns, such as Bilston in the Black Country, had assumed they would be spared. However, due to increasing industrialisation and improved transport links, few towns and villages in that part of the country were far from a canal or waterway. Bilston's population had swelled to around 14,500, thanks to the nearby deposits of iron, coal and limestone then in huge demand. The town's infrastructure was fragile and the only water source, Bilston Brook, had become an open sewer, 'the receptacle of all manner of impurities and loathsome filth disseminating disease and death in all directions.' [85]

Bilston's new accessibility meant that in July 1832 it had been inundated by at least a thousand people attending the Bilston Wake, part of the traditional annual Wakes Week celebrations. The festival originated in the Middle Ages, when local villagers would keep a vigil at the graves of their dead on the eve of 6 November, St Leonard's Day. The practice decreased in popularity after the Reformation and, over the passage of time, Wakes Week became a more secular celebration, with sporting contests and attractions similar to those at fairs and fêtes. Not only did it move location from the churchyard to Bilston's market square, but the date was also changed to midsummer. [86]

The influx of people from surrounding areas, was to prove disastrous for Bilston in the summer of 1832. Elsewhere cholera was already established and the Wakes Week visitors brought the disease with them, tainting Bilston's water supply and infecting the indigenous population. When cholera swept through the town in August and September, 745 died – around one in twenty of the population. [87] Such was the speed at which the disease struck, Bilston could not keep up with burials and cart loads of coffins had to be brought in from Birmingham. [88]

No area of Britain was to be spared from cholera. At this time, the journey by sea from Sunderland to London took only three days, [89] and it is likely that in this way – though no doubt also progressing along the waterways, and via those travelling on foot – that cholera arrived in the capital. The first case in London was attributed to a seaman on board a vessel from Limerick in Ireland, where cholera had broken out the previous August. In the first week of February 1832, when cholera was still confined to Sunderland, Newcastle and Edinburgh, the seaman died in the capital's St Katharine Docks; *The Times* declared, 'The pestilence is among us.'[90]

The following week, seven cases were noted in the riverside areas of Rotherhithe and Limehouse, and then the disease escalated along the River Thames to Southwark and Lambeth on the south bank and to Chelsea. It broke out in Whitechapel in the east, then Westminster and Marylebone. It struck in St Giles, to the east of today's Barbican, and St Luke's in Islington and then throughout the East End: to Bethnal Green, Stepney and Spitalfields. Cholera then broke out in Wandsworth, Woolwich, Blackfriars, the Tower of London, and Millbank Penitentiary.

Millbank was a repository for prisoners who were to be transported to Australia. From here they were sent by barge to the hulks at Woolwich and Chatham, decommissioned naval vessels and merchant ships, many of which had served in the Napoleonic Wars. The hulks were insanitary wooden shells, devoid of their original rigging, sinister spectres moored in the Thames and Medway Estuaries. Unsurprisingly it was at Chatham that cholera next broke out, on the hulks and in the town, then along the Kent coast to Sittingbourne, Faversham, Broadstairs, and up the River Stour to Canterbury. Sheerness was also affected, though an additional source of infection in this area may have been ships quarantined at nearby Stangate Creek.

In July 1832 cholera reached the West Country, arriving first at the port in Plymouth and then flaring up in Exeter. It was rumoured that cholera had been brought to the city by a woman who had nursed a victim in Plymouth; within a day of her return to Exeter she and her two children were suffering from the disease.[91] As in every other town and city in the country, the working population of Exeter were particularly vulnerable to the disease, living in tightly packed houses with poor sanitation. The physician Thomas Shapter chronicled the outbreak in *The History of the Cholera in Exeter in 1832*. He described the living conditions for the poorest in the city thus:

> '... dwellings occupied by from five to fifteen families,
> huddled together in dirty rooms with every offensive

*accompaniment; of slaughter houses in the Butcher-row,*
*with their putrid heaps of offal; of pigs in large numbers*
*kept throughout the City ... of poultry kept in confined*
*cellars and outhouses; of dung-heaps everywhere ... one*
*courtlage [backyard] was visited in which the accumulated*
*filth and soil of thirteen years was deposited'*[92]

Even in the wealthier areas of Exeter, the recently constructed sewers had not been well designed. The water supply, whether for drainage or consumption, was simply not sufficient for the numbers of people who had moved into the city. Whilst many households had access to underground wells, the only public supply of water came from a single source: the ancient conduit by the Hall of the Vicars Choral in South Street, not far from the cathedral. Drinking water was also available from public pumps, but the supply was unreliable. Some citizens collected water from the River Exe or local streams, while others relied on carriers who brought river water into the city in cask-laden carts.[93]

The first case of cholera in Exeter occurred on 18 July 1832, but the authorities initially denied that the disease had arrived in the city, perhaps concerned by the responsibilities they now faced under the new Cholera Prevention Act. Not only did they need to keep on top of the escalating situation, but costs had to be met from local poor rates which they feared would not be sufficient. In Exeter, as noted by historian Norman Longmate, 'money ... was pooled in a central fund for the whole city and spent where needed.'[94]

As cholera spread through Exeter, rumours circulated that medical attendants were proliferating the disease as they went from one person to the next. The citizens became unruly, but the disorder was fuelled in part by drunkenness. Shapter compared the atmosphere to the days of the plague and claimed that the drunken state of the Exeter's 'lower orders' was 'induced, not only by the general excitement prevailing, but by an idea that brandy was a preventative and panacea for the Cholera.'[95] A further 1,135 citizens were to suffer from cholera in Exeter, of a population of 28,242, and approximately 345 died.[96]

In Britain, between 1831 and 1832, at least 32,000 people

succumbed to the disease.[97] Prior to the formal registration of deaths, which began in 1837, it is impossible to be precise and parish registers rarely record the cause of death. Some believe 32,000 to be an underestimate and that perhaps more than 50,000 perished.[98] Brandy was not the cure for cholera that many had hoped, and physicians were well aware of this, including a young Dr John Snow, who urged temperance at Pateley Bridge, North Yorkshire in 1836:

> *'I feel it my duty to endeavour to convince you of the physical evils sustained to your health by using intoxicating liquors even in the greatest moderation ... The brandy treatment has been extensively tried in cholera, but it is now abandoned in all parts of the world. If the debility is not so great that life is not destroyed by it (brandy), still it hurries on and makes more violent that reaction, that secondary fever which is most to be dreaded, and increases the tendency which there is to inflammation in the head and elsewhere. The common practice of applying to these drinks when chilled with cold, is equally injurious. It generally makes worse if it does not altogether bring on all the ill effects usually attributed to the cold.'[99]*

Brandy continued to be advertised as a cure for many diseases, including cholera, for years to come, no doubt boosting the profits of J.T. Betts and Company. Brandy was equalled in its efficacy by other remedies, which were widely advertised in the press, alongside recipes for various medicinal mixtures, (as was discussed in Chapter 1). By the late 1840s, doctors were coming to the conclusion that electricity might be the solution. Observers in Paris noticed that the amount of electricity they could measure in the air varied and at times when these quantities were lower, the incidence of cholera increased.[100] Then, when doctors in London subjected a dying child to a pulse of electricity, they were astonished to observe that she rallied, and it was believed that the French may have made a major discovery.[101]

In 1848 a small advertisement was printed in *The Times* for 'patent self-cleansing filters' to purify water: 'Dr. Strickland has reason to believe that unhealthy weather renders cistern water to a certain extent unwholesome, and decidedly recommends, especially for delicate persons and children, the purification of water by filtration just before using or drinking it.' [102] At a cost of 8 shillings and sixpence, these filters would have made a far greater impact during the cholera outbreaks to follow later in the century. Yet, as brandy was cheaper and far more palatable, the advertisement had little impact.

# CHAPTER 3

# The Wretched State of the Poor:
# The influence of politics and philosophy
# on the living and sanitary conditions
# of the poor

The poverty that existed in nineteenth century Britain and the deplorable conditions in which working people lived are hard to imagine today. There was no clean running water and sewage discharged freely into open drains, streams and rivers. Household waste was not collected regularly, mice and rats were a constant presence, as was the threat of disease. So many of the conveniences that make our modern world clean, healthy and pleasant were absent, and in the towns and cities the stench must have been overwhelming.

Throughout the nineteenth century, levels of migration increased from a largely depressed and impoverished countryside to towns and cities, where many hoped to find prosperity and more lucrative employment. For most this was not to be the case and, as migration increased, living conditions for the urban working poor became more crowded and unhealthy.

Today factors associated with urban living, such as air pollution, are understood to have a detrimental impact on health,[1] but in the crowded cities of Victorian Britain, this was only part of the problem. Density of housing, poor sanitation, carbon and chemical emissions from homes and factories all combined to shorten life expectancy. In addition, without the vote or the right to form trades unions, the working population had no democratic representation or a means for change.[2]

By 1850, the population of Britain had grown to over 18 million[3] – a rise of 12 million in a single century – and for the first time in history the urban population outnumbered the rural. The 1851 Census revealed that 54 per cent of the population lived in towns and cities.[4] Demographic change was particularly evident in industrialised areas such as the north, the Midlands and London. In the capital, between 1840 and 1900 the population swelled from 800,000 to 7,000,000.[4] During the first decades of the nineteenth century, when cholera had first visited Britain's shores, some migrants had started to fare better in the towns but for most life continued to be a struggle – a situation that would take considerable time to improve. Some years later, in 1891, John Atkinson Hobson noted in his *Problems of Poverty* that:

> ' ... *out of an estimated population of some 38,000,000, only 11,000,000, or about three out of every ten persons in the richest country in Europe, belong to a class which is able to live in decent comfort, free from the pressing cares of a close economy. The other seven are of necessity confined to a standard of life little, if at all, above the line of bare necessaries.*'[5]

Population density in the towns and cities was a serious issue for public health. Urban living conditions provided the perfect crucible for certain infectious diseases, such as tuberculosis, which flourished in damp, unventilated, densely packed dwellings and was far more prevalent in the town than the country. The most vulnerable were the working poor, who were under nourished and had little resistance to disease. In 1831 as Britain braced itself for cholera (as discussed in the previous chapter), many in the medical community had already identified a connection between poverty and disease, and understood the susceptibility of the working poor, as the physician Sir Gilbert Blaine commented:

> '*It is found that the squalid population do, by their filth, stench, bad clothing, bad and scanty diet, and other constituents of misery, not only contract and harbour*

*infection, but attract it as it were ... When the Court left London on occasion of the last plague in 1665, the Lord Chancellor Clarendon, who accompanied them, relates in the history of his own life, that the calamity had fallen almost exclusively on the miserable and indigent.'*[6]

Statistical results from the 1841 Census gave Registrar General William Farr an opportunity to examine in greater detail mortality rates in England and Wales for the whole population, (as discussed in Chapter 5). He compiled life tables, showing that life expectancy was considerable lower in urban environments: 37 for men living in London and just 26 for those in Liverpool, nearly two decades lower than the average of 45 in rural Surrey.[7]

When epidemic cholera broke out in the North East of Britain in 1831, (as discussed in the previous chapter), its first victims were the poor who lived closest to the water's edge, in squalid, insanitary housing. As the disease spread, the poor continued to fall victim to it. Cholera will infect the most vulnerable first, but not exclusively, as the citizens of York discovered. Cholera is more likely to strike those living in insanitary conditions who do not prepare their food hygienically and neglect to wash their hands before eating. The disease is also more deadly for those weakened by other diseases and infections: pregnant women and those with low levels of stomach acid, including the poorly nourished and those who drink alcohol regularly.

Until very recently, it was believed that considerable numbers of pathogenic cholera bacteria needed to be ingested to start the cycle of infection, yet the work of molecular biologist Professor Bonnie L. Bassler has shown that this is not the case, (as discussed in Chapter 2). The main implication of this discovery is that hygiene behaviour is a key factor for infection, as evidenced by the way in which cholera struck down more affluent members of society in the later epidemics of the nineteenth century.

As with many infectious diseases, greater susceptibility is caused by an ignorance of how to prevent oral-faecal infection. This is still an issue today, not just in developing countries but also in Britain, where research has revealed that the public is surprisingly ignorant of the importance of good hand hygiene. The work of Dr Val Curtis of the Hygiene Centre at the London School of Hygiene and Tropical Medicine has shown that clean hands and hygienic food preparation are as important as clean water in disease prevention:

> ' ... *promotion of safe hygiene is the single most cost-effective means of preventing infectious disease, investment in hygiene is low both in the health and in the water and sanitation sectors. Evidence shows the benefit of improved hygiene, especially for improved handwashing and safe stool disposal.*'[8]

Moreover, Dr Curtis and her colleagues have demonstrated in their work that washing your hands with soap can reduce the risk of diarrhoeal disease by 42 to 47 per cent.[9]

The poorest areas of Britain's Victorian towns and cities were those clustered around rivers, canals and estuaries – the main transportation arteries before the building of the railways began in the 1830s. Here many industrial works were also located, which depended on a plentiful supply of water for new manufacturing processes fuelled by steam power. By 1801 London was already the largest city in Western Europe with a population of almost one million.[10] In the first half of the nineteenth century, the areas of the city worst affected by cholera were on the banks of the River Thames: in Southwark (in the parishes of St Saviour's, St Olave's, and St George's); Bermondsey; Newington St Mary; Lambeth; Wandsworth; Camberwell; and Rotherhithe.[11] By the 1840s, these areas were densely populated with tenement buildings, which had been speedily erected at the lowest possible cost for workers and their families. Those on the southern banks of the Thames were constructed on marshland; built cheek by jowl, they were damp, poorly ventilated and possessed little or no sanitation.

Overcrowding was not just a problem in London but also across Britain's towns and cities. It is perhaps unsurprising that life expectancy was lowest in Liverpool, as the number of people per dwelling within the city had risen from 6.4 in 1831 to 6.9 in 1841, and by this time a quarter of the population lived in back-to-back terraced houses sharing a common rear wall. In Nottingham, Birmingham and Leeds around 65 to 70 per cent of houses were built in the same fashion. Accessed from a court or street, most consisted of a single room on each floor, connected by a stairway.[12]

By the 1840s Britain's urban population had risen to an alarming level, with 138,000 persons per square mile in Liverpool, 100,000 in Manchester, 87,000 in Leeds, and 50,000 in London.[13] The figure for London seems small in comparison but it is a city-wide average and does not take into account specific areas. For example, in the St Giles area from 1841 to 1847, 27 of the district's dwellings (comprising five rooms each) increased occupancy from 655 to 1,095. In just six years the average number of people occupying a single building rose from 24 to over 40.[14]

To save money, families and strangers cohabited in single rooms, and whole tenement blocks and back-to back houses shared a handful of outside privies. Privies drained into cesspits, which were rarely emptied, while open sewers, drains and ditches were prone to overflow during heavy rain and at high tide in riverside areas. Access to tenements like those on the south banks of the Thames was usually through muddy, narrow alleys. Dwellings and factories occupied the same spaces and were built around courtyards, which were often also occupied by slaughterhouses and piggeries. Pigs and cows were typically kept in enclosures, not just in courtyards but also on street corners, mimicking rural practices, and in London pigs were often kept in cellars (as discussed in the previous chapter).

Rubbish was infrequently collected from the streets and in areas such as Lambeth, on the low-lying south bank of the River Thames huge refuse piles, which in some cases rose to the first floors of the buildings, were a familiar sight. Flooding in these riverside areas caused muck to mix freely with human and animal effluent, and in the warm summer months flies and mosquitoes proliferated, alongside rats and mice.

Houses had no running water and many poor riverside areas, such as those in Exeter and London, lacked stand pipes, forcing residents to take their water from the rivers by bucket.[15] Yet those streets with communal standpipes fared no better, as the water provided came from the very same source: the river. By the middle of the century, in London and most other densely populated towns and cities, the rivers had become open sewers. Of the situation in Bristol, Dr William Budd remarked:

> *'There was a striking contrast between rich and poor. The latter lived for the most part in a series of wretched tenements built around courtyards, each with a single tap and three privies which discharged directly into the river. It is not surprising that the cholera epidemic of 1831-2 took a terrible toll among the poor.'* [16]

The first act of parliament designed to address the infrastructure of metropolitan areas was the Metropolitan Buildings Act of 1844. Schedule H of the act was concerned with the improved building of drains and the connection to sewers, however the new requirements related only to structures built after 1 January 1845, and as an amendment to the bill specified, only if the sewer was positioned within 100 feet of any new building. Whilst this was a move in the right direction, the legislation did not go nearly far enough.[17] An amendment in 1847 included the requirement for cesspools and privies to empty into a drain or sewer,[18] but improvements were slow and difficult to enforce.

The filth in towns and cities and the threat of infectious diseases such as cholera prompted the passing of local legislation and bills, including the 1842 Leeds Improvements Act and the 1846 Liverpool Sanitary Act, continued the move towards better sanitation. The latter is regarded by many, including social historian Eric Midwinter, to be the 'first piece of comprehensive Health [sic] legislation passed in England. It made the Town Council responsible for drainage, paving, sewerage and cleaning, it permitted the appointment of a Borough Engineer, an Inspector of Nuisance and the first-ever Medical Officer of Health.'[19]

In 1847 Liverpool appointed James Newlands as Borough Engineer[20] and Dr William Henry Duncan as the city's first Medical Officer. Together they did much to improve sanitation and public health in

Liverpool, with new initiatives such as rubbish collection, street cleaning, public bath houses and the provision of clean water. Subsequent legislation aided progress, as did Newlands' integrated sewer system, the first of its kind.[21]

Three successive Nuisances Removal and Diseases Prevention Acts of 1846, 1848 and 1849 gave local authorities the power to investigate, remove or disinfect so-called nuisances, and areas of human habitation deemed detrimental to health and capable of encouraging the spread of disease. The legislation defined a nuisance as a 'foul and offensive ditch, gutter, drain, privy, cesspool, or ash-pit ... swine, or any accumulation of dung, manure, offal, filth, refuse ... kept so as to be a nuisance to or injurious to the health of any person.' [22]

The 1846 Nuisances Removal Act was also known as the 'Cholera Bill', as it was put in place to facilitate prevention of the disease. During the 1848-9 cholera outbreak the legislation was deemed helpful for the General Board of Health, but in urban areas, and especially in the tenements of London's poorest parishes, little changed. The huge scale of the task, the cost of improvements and a lack of effective management prevented most local authorities from taking immediate action.

In 1847 the Metropolitan Sanitary Commission was appointed to 'inquire whether any, and what, special means might be requisite for the improvement of the health of the metropolis, with regard more especially to the better house, street and land drainage.'[23]

Sanitary reform was essential, yet in London progress was impeded by the existence of eight separate bodies all with their own boards. Each board had a responsibility to its local area, but their work was autonomous, with little communication between them and no uniformity; even the sizes of drains could differ from parish to parish.[24]

Lord John Russell's Whig government appointed Lord Morpeth as chairman to the Metropolitan Sanitary Commission, along with 21 other chief officers, including Edwin Chadwick, Dr Thomas Southwood Smith and the Health of Towns commissioner, Richard Owen.[25] The Commission's priority was to highlight the locations where cholera was most likely to occur in future. Work began in September 1847 and the First Report presented the following year. It included evidence compiled by separate Sanitary Committees from the London parishes, who had been sent to the poorest areas, where living conditions and sanitation were of the worst. The conclusion of the Metropolitan Sanitary Commission was that cholera was contagious. Convinced that insanitary living conditions were inextricably linked to the spread of diseases such as cholera, Edwin Chadwick felt that the cleansing and removal of nuisances would be desirable. His solution, which would incur high costs and cause upheaval, was most fiercely opposed by Sir William Pym, Superintendent of Quarantine at the Privy Council Office, who strongly advised Chadwick against taking such action.[26]

The Commission's findings resulted in the passing of the 1848 Metropolitan Sewers Act. It paved the way for the creation of the first Metropolitan Commission of Sewers, which employed the same members as had been appointed to the Metropolitan Sanitary Commission the previous year, and who replaced over a thousand district commissioners.[27] Headed by Lord Morpeth, the Commission included members with a wide range of experience: Lord Ebrington; Joseph Hume; R.A. Slaney M.P.; Dr Neil Arnott; Dr Thomas Southwood Smith; Professor Richard Owen; Sir James Clark, physician to Queen Victoria; Sir Henry de la Beche, Director General of the Ordnance Survey; the Rev W. Stone, the Dean of Westminster; philanthropists Sir Edward Buxton and John Bullar; John Walter III, the proprietor of *The Times*; Lord Ashley; and Edwin Chadwick himself.[28] The new authority that emerged, the Metropolitan Commission of Sewers, appointed Joseph Bazalgette as Assistant Surveyor.

The 1848 Metropolitan Sewers Act extended previous legislation to existing buildings, requiring the owners to construct toilet facilities. Commissioners were also given the power to order the connection of buildings to sewers. An 1849 amendment further extended these powers to improve drainage, passing the cost on to the property owner.[29] In London there were six Metropolitan Sewers Commissions from 1848 to 1855. An initial survey of the city's sewers was attempted by the Ordnance Survey, but progress was slow and hampered by legal problems. Waste was still being flushed into the Thames and, as the miasmatists still refused to believe cholera was waterborne, a new sewer system was not perceived as such an urgent a priority as the cleansing of noxious domestic facilities.

The Second Commission in 1849 appointed some additional members: Sir John Burgoyne; Captain Vetch, of the Tidal Harbour Commission; Captain Dawson, of the Ordnance Survey; and Cuthbert Johnson, a manure expert. The health reform campaigner Henry Austin, the husband of Charles Dickens's sister Letitia, was also appointed to the Commission as a consulting engineer.[30] He suggested that sewage should be collected in reservoirs and then pumped out of the capital for agricultural use. Other plans were considered but no agreement was reached, and so in August 1849, following Bazalgette's appointment as Assistant Surveyor, an invitation was issued requesting other engineers to submit suggestions.[31]

Each Commission suffered from disagreement and lack of progress. The Third Commission began in October 1849, and included the railway engineers Robert Stephenson and Frank Forster, as well as a new Assistant Surveyor named Edward Cresy. By August 1850, none of the schemes hitherto suggested was judged worth acting on, and so Forster was asked to create something new. His response would form the basis of Bazalgette's final design for London's new sewer system (discussed in greater detail in Chapter 8).

Forster came from Newcastle and had worked with Robert Stephenson on the building of the London and Birmingham and Chester and Holyhead railways. With a background in mining engineering, he had also taken part in a project on the coalfield in Richmond, Virginia in the United States. Forster had some formidable experience, but the Second Commission was a more daunting task than all the rest, and his obituary was to hint that it led to his untimely death in April 1852: 'Worn out by annoyances, Mr. Forster resigned his appointment, and died a few weeks afterwards.'[32]

With costs escalating, the Third Commission resigned and a Fourth was appointed between July and October 1852, with Bazalgette in Forster's place as Engineer to the Commission. During the Fourth and Fifth Commissions, Bazalgette continued to work on his sewer plans. His priority in 1852 was the construction of drains for the streets and houses of London which would all empty into the River Thames. By 1854, Bazalgette had completed his design, having re-worked Forster's ideas. Together with the engineer William Haywood, who had also collaborated with Forster, Bazalgette presented the plan to Robert Stephenson and William Cubitt, who both gave their approval.[33]

Arguments over costs continued and objections to Bazalgette's proposals emerged from the General Board of Health and Edwin Chadwick, who had left office at the end of the Second Commission. The Fifth Commission thus resigned and the Sixth and last commenced in November 1854. Following further outbreaks of cholera in 1848-9 and 1853-4, the urgency of the situation had been felt for some time and, in the hope of injecting new energy into the process, the Sixth Commission also included representatives from each of the Metropolitan Boroughs. In January 1855 it was agreed to begin the building of the scheme as originally set out by Forster, but this was soon thwarted due to a problem with the purchase of the land required.[34]

The Metropolitan Sewers Commissions were the forerunners of the Metropolitan Board of Works, which was set up in 1853. Only after the Board had been established would any real progress be made on the building of London's new sewage system.

The urgent need to overhaul London's infrastructure was mirrored across Britain's towns and cities. Caused by the shift in the nineteenth century from an agrarian to an industrial society, this occurred for a number of reasons. By the 1830s the mechanisation of farming processes had caused the decline of many traditional jobs and skills. The enclosure and consolidation of open spaces at the end of the eighteenth century meant that agricultural labourers were no longer able to cultivate common land or graze their livestock on it. In addition, the old practices of seasonal hiring and the lodging of agricultural labourers were being phased out by new farm owners. War with France and the revolutions taking place there and in America also took a toll upon Britain, forcing political change and speeding up the move towards greater mechanisation.

Restrictions on trade during the Napoleonic Wars affected corn prices, but when the conflict ended in 1815 prices fell rapidly. In an attempt to protect the domestic market, the Corn Laws were passed in parliament to prohibit the importation of cheap foreign grain. Whilst this was beneficial for landowners, the legislation meant that people now had to pay more for their bread. In addition to this, a series of bad harvests affected the supply of grain and other crops, while in Ireland the repeated failure of the potato harvest from the mid-1840s caused famine and mass migration, adding to the overcrowding of Britain's growing towns and cities.

Riots were not uncommon at this time, and the Government feared mass insurrection. To alleviate the distress of the poor in the countryside, the Speenhamland System of topping up workers' wages when bread prices rose – first implemented in Berkshire during the 1790s – became more widely adopted. The amount spent on poor relief increased from just under £2 million in 1783-4 to around £7 million in 1820-21.[35] Unrest was rife and the need for social reform became more and more apparent. Despite the passing of the Reform Act in 1832 and the hope for greater representation in parliament, working men and their middle class supporters continued to set up societies and associations such as trades unions, which were finally legalised in 1825.

In February 1832 Earl Grey's Whig government appointed a Royal Commission to look into the way in which financial relief was administered to the poor in local parishes in England and Wales, and whether such methods could be improved upon.[36] Named The Poor Law Inquiry Commission, it was overseen by the Bishop of London, Charles Blomfield, and its nine members included the political economist and lawyer, Nassau Senior. Senior was of the view that the key to eradicating poverty was to improve the provision of education and increase productivity. Nassau was a friend of the young Edwin Chadwick, whom he appointed as an Assistant to the Commission.

The committee drew up two questionnaires for rural areas and one for towns. However, the response was poor and so it was decided to send out 26 newly appointed Assistant Commissioners, who would be left to decide for themselves whom and where to visit, as it was impossible to go to every parish in the short time allotted. As a result, only about 3,000 locations were visited – around a fifth of all local authorities. Such was the haste and inefficiency of its compilation that much of the 1834 Poor Law Report was written before all of the evidence had been received,[37] and its contents reflected to a large extent the views of Edwin Chadwick.[38]

The commissioners believed that the old system of poor relief and not the paupers themselves should be blamed for their dependence upon the state. The old system, as they saw it, also offered little encouragement for the labouring classes to restrain the size of their families, as parishes offered greater help to those with more children. It enabled farm owners to keep wages low, as their workers were subsidised by the local parishes, which in some cases included rent. The effect was often a rise in poor rates and a decline in labour productivity.[39]

The 1834 *Poor Law Report* concluded:

> *'It appears from all our returns ... that in every district, the discontent of the labouring classes is proportioned to the money dispensed in poor's* [sic] *rates, or in voluntary charities. The able-bodied unmarried labourers are discontented, from being put to a disadvantage as compared with the married. The paupers are discontented from their expectations being raised by the ordinary administration of the system, beyond any means of satisfying them.'* [40]

These findings, suggested that outdoor relief, (as a parish's financial support of its poorer residents was known), needed to be controlled and restricted. The aim of the commissioners, and as they explained in the report, would be to make pauperism as difficult as possible, 'a principle which we find universally admitted ... is that his situation on the whole shall not be made really or apparently so eligible as the situation of the independent labourer of the lowest class.'[41]

The new system was intended to act as a deterrent to people at risk of becoming reliant on outdoor relief, and certain passages in the 1834 report paved the way for a new institution which was to become one of the most feared places, the workhouse: '... all relief whatever to able-bodied persons or to their families, otherwise in well-regulated workhouses (i.e., places where they may be set to work ... ) shall be declared unlawful and shall cease.'[42]

The workhouses were to be funded by the local parish or union, which would be overseen by a central board to ensure uniformity. The new rules also excluded the mothers of illegitimate children from claiming financial support from the fathers, 'unless their identity could be proven,' and all children would be deemed independent of their mother's settlement at the age of 16.[43]

The new bill enshrining these measures in law, The Poor Law Amendment Act, was passed in August 1834, and in its wake created a new Poor Law Board staffed by commissioners, which was based at Somerset House in London. The bill was not as clear as it might have been and, whilst it required the commissioners to use the *Poor Law Report* as their guide, its practical implementation was left to their own discretion. There was much resistance to the new law, particularly in the north of England, where an anti-Poor Law movement began. Indeed in 1847, the Board was replaced by a new body, led by a member of parliament who could be held accountable to the electorate.

The new Poor Law did not make life better or easier for the most impoverished members of British society and the workhouse was greatly feared. Rather than providing an environment in which the poor could rebuild their lives and make a fresh start, the workhouse separated families and became a place of deprivation and abuse (as will be demonstrated in Chapter 4).

As is evidenced by the list of those selected for the first Metropolitan Commission of Sewers, the men who sat on the different Royal Commissions in the nineteenth century were from a variety of professions. However, most had similar backgrounds and some were friends who held shared beliefs on how to shape society. Amongst this circle of London's elite were many of the surgeons and physicians who had studied at Edinburgh University.

The teaching of the Theory and Practice of Medicine had begun at Edinburgh in 1720 and the university's School of Medicine had opened six years later under the first Chair of Anatomy, Alexander Monro. At this time Oxford and Cambridge only admitted Anglicans, but at

Edinburgh there were no such restrictions and the university swiftly became a magnet for Non-conformists. Free, liberal thinking was encouraged and progressive teaching was the norm, particularly under Professor of Moral Philosophy Dugald Stewart, and later Professor of Medicine William Pulteney Alison, the Scottish Poor Law reformer.

In the second half of the eighteenth century Scotland had developed a much closer relationship with France, both in terms of trade and ideas, and Edinburgh became the centre for the Scottish Enlightenment, and as Voltaire noted, '*Nous nous tournons vers l'Écosse pour trouver toutes nos idées sur la civilisation,*' (roughly, 'We look to Scotland to understand civilisation.').[44]

Edinburgh graduates included the surgeons James Phillips Kay-Shuttleworth and Thomas Southwood Smith, who were to shape future legislation, together with barrister Edwin Chadwick and surgeon Neil Arnott. They were also all members of The London Debating Society, where they came under the influence of John Stuart Mill and Jeremy Bentham. In addition, Chadwick was involved with the Political Economy Club and the Philosophical Radicals, which included Bentham, John Stuart Mill and his father James, and the Poor Law Commissioner Nassau Senior.[45]

In 1830 Bentham employed Chadwick to work on the completion of his *Constitutional Code,*[46] and the following year Chadwick moved in with Bentham to work as his literary secretary.[47] The men became close friends. Chadwick had been brought up in a liberal non-conformist family in Manchester, and his father, James, was a radical journalist, a friend of the famous political activist Thomas Paine,[48] whose ideas had inspired the American revolutionaries. During his early years in London as a legal apprentice, Chadwick supported himself by writing articles for the press, focusing on the state of London's poor. One of the publications he contributed to was Bentham's *Westminster Review*, which Bentham had founded in 1823 as a voice for the Radicals' cause and the theory of Utilitarianism. The interpretation of this philosophy undoubtedly had an impact on how Chadwick and his circle viewed poverty and how best to help those in need.

Happiness was a central tenet of Bentham's Utilitarianism, along with the importance of making the right choices for as many people as possible. [49] This idea was extended by Mill but with the consequence that morally dubious choices could be justified as long as the overall outcome was beneficial for the majority.[50] Perhaps the introduction of the workhouse as a deterrent, and the ensuing misery this caused, can be explained by Utilitarian views. However, historian Christopher Hamlin believes Chadwick's approach was of a broader nature: 'His poor law was derived from the axioms of political economy, which were in turn based on universal laws of human nature. Correct application of these laws and axioms guaranteed social harmony.' [51]

A confirmed miasmatist, Chadwick was convinced that the health of the poorest in society was linked to their living conditions, and if these could be improved then the poor would be far less dependent on the state. Following his initial appointment to the Poor Law Inquiry Commission as an Assistant, Chadwick became Secretary to the Poor Law Commission from 1834 to 1847. However, in 1833 he also worked for the Royal Commission on factories, which was concerned with the treatment of children working in industry. This led to the Factory Act of the same year, which not only limited the hours children were allowed to work but also introduced some schooling for children under the age of 13. [52] Chadwick's influence on this legislation is also seen in the introduction of inspectors, who were responsible to Government and had the power to enforce the law with penalties.

Chadwick's associate James Phillips Kay-Shuttleworth had been an Assistant Poor Law Commissioner for Suffolk and Norfolk. He was firmly of the belief that education was the key to eradicating the problems associated with poverty but, like Chadwick, he also understood the connection with disease. Kay's 1832 work, *The Moral and Physical Condition of the Working Classes Employed in the Cotton Manufacture in Manchester*, shaped the thinking of other social reformers, including Friedrich Engels who drew on Kay's work in his 1845 study, *The Condition of the Working Class in England*.

In 1837 Kay-Shuttleworth had been appointed by the Poor Law Board to look into the state of the weavers in Spitalfields who, even when in full employment, were not receiving a living wage. The work was conducted with another of Chadwick's circle, Neil Arnott, a former East India Company ship's surgeon, who had a great interest in cholera and sanitation; in 1843 he became a member of the Health of Towns Commission.[53] Kay-Shuttleworth and Arnott worked together again in 1838, examining conditions in the East End of London at Wapping, Ratcliff and Stepney.[54]

Another of this tight group of friends and colleagues, Edinburgh alumnus Thomas Southwood Smith worked at the London Fever Hospital, the Eastern Dispensary and the Jews' Hospital in Whitechapel. At the same time as Kay-Shuttleworth and Arnott were working in the East End of London, he was invited by the Poor Law Commission to investigate conditions in the same area, in Bethnal Green and Stepney. He produced a paper, entitled *On some of the physical causes of sickness and mortality to which the poor are particularly exposed and which are capable of removal by sanitary regulations, exemplified in the present condition of the Bethnal Green and Whitechapel districts, as ascertained by personal inspection.* His work backed up Kay-Shuttleworth's observations on the cotton mills of Manchester, linking disease to living conditions and emphasising the need for good sanitation;[55] both sets of research were presented as appendices to the annual *Poor Law Report.*[56]

Following the publication of this latest report in 1838 and its appendices, the Bishop of London, Charles Blomfield, who had sat on the Poor Law Commission in 1832, asked in the House of Lords for an inquiry into the sanitary conditions of the working classes to be undertaken. However, just as the 1831 cholera outbreak had roused the authorities from complacency, a response to Blomfield came in 1837-8, as London suffered severe outbreaks of influenza and typhus fever. Seizing the moment, Chadwick, then Secretary to the Poor Law Commissioners, once again put forward his views to the government on the direct link between disease and poverty, and so forcible was his argument that it was finally agreed to undertake a study to analyse the connection.

In 1838 the Poor Law Commissioners began the inquiry that would culminate in the 1842 *Report on the Sanitary Condition of the Labouring Population.*[57] In this report Chadwick would make his ethos clear: 'In the great mass of cases in every part of the country, in the rural districts and in the places of commercial pressure, the attacks of disease are upon those in full employment, the attack of fever precedes the destitution, not destitution the disease.'[58]

The 1842 report covered England, Wales and Scotland and Chadwick worked systematically, gathering evidence by writing to assistant Poor Law commissioners, local officers and guardians, and statisticians such as William Farr and Charles Babbage.[59] The completed report discussed in detail the deplorable living and sanitary conditions of the labouring classes, including categories covering drainage, street and road cleansing, water supplies, ventilation, over-crowding and the predisposing causes of disease. It also looked at health and life expectancy and the economic state of the working poor. The report finally considered the cost of housing improvements for tenants and owners, and the responsibility of employers to provide better conditions for workers and live-in employees. It even included a note on the beneficial effect of 'public walks and gardens on the health and morals of the lower classes of the population of the environment.'[60]

The overriding aim of the report was to establish a link between poor living conditions and disease, but the main obstacle to Chadwick's proposals was cost. However, such was the concern by the other Poor Law Commissioners over the controversial content and nature of the report, it was agreed to publish it only in Chadwick's name. Determined to make the work known, Chadwick ordered a privately printed quarto version which he advertised in the press and sent to influential friends. The report was an important factor in the government's appointment of a Royal Commission on the Health of Towns in 1843. Chaired by Chadwick, members included his associates, Arnott and Southwood Smith.[61]

The Royal Commission presented its evidence in 1844 and 1845, making the recommendation that central government should take responsibility for public health and oversee the regulation of sanitary condition in urban areas. It also urged a complete reform for the regulation of sanitation and the creation of a single administrative body.[62]

At the time, there were several other independent groups and societies exerting pressure for change and a reform in legislation to help the poor. Amongst these was the Society for Improving the

Condition of the Labouring Classes, founded by Lord Shaftesbury and Robert Benton Seeley in 1844, with Prince Albert as President.[63] Also established in 1844 was the Health of Towns Association, by Chadwick's colleague Southwood Smith. Supported by many of the great influential social reformers of the day, such as Lord Ashley and Lord Normanby, the association exerted considerable influence.[64] At its public meetings members of the medical profession were invited to speak and books and pamphlets were circulated.[65]

Whilst pressure groups had an impact, the Poor Law Commission was abolished in 1847, mainly as a result of the Andover Workhouse scandal. The appalling conditions in workhouses like Andover will be discussed further in the next chapter, but here the situation was particularly severe. Costs were kept to a minimum, inmates suffered from a lack of food and they were subjected to a strict and unpleasant work regime, which included the arduous crushing of bones for fertiliser. Inmates were so hungry that many of them ripped scraps from the very bones they were given to crush. Everyone connected with Andover was found to be at fault, including the Poor Law Commissioners who had not dealt with the deteriorating situation.[66] The Poor Law Commission was replaced in 1847 by the Poor Law Board, which hitherto would be directly accountable to parliament.[67]

However, once again the threat and fear of infectious disease would prompt further change when cholera broke out in 1848. The disease followed a similar path as the 1831-2 epidemic, emerging in June in Russia, before sweeping across Europe. By September it had reached Germany and France,[68] but possible cases had already been reported in Britain before its arrival was established in the autumn.[69] On 31 August 1848, The Public Health Act was passed, establishing a Central Board of Health for the next five years. This enabled local boards of health to be set up in England and Wales, but not in London, where perhaps there was the greatest need. A clause in the new legislation stipulated that in the capital a board could only be set up 'either when petitioned by not less than one tenth of the taxpayers or compulsorily when the average mortality rate over a period of seven years exceeded 23 per 1,000.'[70]

Chadwick took up the post of Public Health Commissioner in

September 1848, working with Lord Morpeth, Lord Ashley, and later Southwood Smith.[71] Local boards were given responsibility for water, sewage, the cleaning of streets, the removal of nuisances and the regulation of cemeteries and slaughterhouses.[72] In order to oversee these responsibilities, each local board was to appoint an officer of health from the medical profession, an inspector of nuisances, a surveyor, a treasurer and a clerk.[73]

The establishment of the Board of Health was a turning point, but it by no means resolved the condition of the labouring poor, particularly as it did not allow local boards in London. Elsewhere progress was impeded by the Board's inability to overcome local opposition to reform, comparisons to the mistakes made by the Poor Law Commission, and Chadwick's personal inflexibility.[74]

In July 1854 Chadwick's position was abolished and the Board was reconstituted and made responsible to parliament.[75] A new era began with the appointment of Dr John Simon as Chief Medical Officer in 1855, a position he held for three years. Simon had previously been the first Medical Officer of Health for the City of London – the second such appointment in the country after Dr William Henry Duncan in Liverpool. Chadwick retired on a £1,000 per annum pension and was knighted in 1889.[76]

Conditions for the labouring poor were not to change for very many years, and comprehensive, free health care would only become available to all with the establishment of the National Health Service after the Second World War. Improvements to urban infrastructure, including sanitation, were made in the second half of the nineteenth century, yet up until the 1960s and beyond working people continued to live in polluted, densely populated urban environments, in tenement or terraced houses with only cold running water and outside lavatories.

Had politics and philosophy not got in the way, perhaps greater progress might have been made to improve living and sanitary conditions for the working poor during the nineteenth century. The words of Bartholomew Peter Drouet who ran a children's workhouse in Tooting, South London (whose story is told in the following chapter) may best describe the problem. The treatment of the working poor during this period, he said, was 'an experiment.'[77]

# CHAPTER 4

# Cholera and Tooting's Pauper Paradise: Workhouse conditions and how cholera devastated a children's institution

The story of the Infant Pauper Asylum at Tooting in south-west London illustrates how the most vulnerable members of society, pauper children, were treated under the Poor Law system set up in 1834. Later dubbed by Charles Dickens as 'The Paradise at Tooting, or The Tooting Farm', this children's workhouse was established in 1804. The horrors that took place there during the 1848-9 cholera outbreak were revealed ten years after Dickens had published *Oliver Twist*, his indictment of the treatment of children in the workhouse and the new Poor Law system. The establishment at Tooting was taken over by Bartholomew Peter Drouet around 1825, and it was under his management that pauper children from London began to be 'farmed' there.

The sending of children from inner London parishes to the countryside had begun many years before during the eighteenth century, in response to the alarming rise in infant mortality. The social reformer Jonas Hanway was active in promoting a bill in 1767, which became known as Hanway's Act and 'extended the requirement for parishes to maintain and report clear records [of pauper children and] ... that all children below the age of four years should be nursed in the country at least three miles from London and Westminster (five miles in certain circumstances).'[1]

Drouet's, as the institution came to be known, was situated in an old house called Surrey Hall on today's Tooting High Street, on the west side of the road, just north of the junction with Garratt Lane.[2] Surrey Hall was a former old family mansion, with many outbuildings, on a

79

plot of some 52 acres, most of which had been given up for agricultural use. In 1849 the establishment housed 1,372 children, not all of whom were orphans but pauper children whose parents were unable to look after them or were themselves in the workhouse. At Drouet's the children were crammed into small, poorly ventilated, filthy dormitories, many of them three to a bed. They were supplied with a pair of uncovered tubs in each room to relieve themselves during the night,[3] and the stench from these tubs was awful, as *The Times* later described: 'when they wet the bed they are put four in a bed as a punishment, and had to lay on a cold oilcloth, with a straw bed underneath ... boys [were] so hungry ... they have [had] ... to eat the stuff out of the pig-tubs and the wash given to the pigs.'[4] The tubs laden with urine and excrement were carted downstairs by the children in the morning to be emptied, then filled with water which was used to wash down the bedroom floors.[5]

The pauper children had been farmed out following the approval of the Poor Law Commissioners in 1847, at a cost to their parish of 4s and 6d per week, with the additional benefit of 'Mr. Drouet's having the labour of the children,'[6] meaning that he was also entitled to the profits from the sale of their work. Children were engaged for long hours in agricultural work; household chores; needlework, including shirt making (some 50 dozen were being produced a week in 1846);[7] and shoe making. For this they were paid a meagre amount, if anything at all.[8] It was later estimated that it cost as little as 2s 6½d to maintain a child each week, leaving Drouet a potential gross profit from 1,372 children of 1s 11½d per week per head – a total of £134 7s 2d per week or £6,986 12s 8d per year.

In the 1841 Census, Drouet is shown living at the institution with his wife Maria (née Fraiser) and half-sister Miriam, but the couple also owned a substantial property by the sea at Margate. In the census 30-year-old Maria, ten years younger than her husband, is listed as 'Matron' and Miriam, aged 15, is noted as 'Assistant Matron' with Sarah Day. Whilst the occupation of the children housed at Drouet's was listed as 'School',[9] in fact they received little education. The single schoolroom meant to house 500 boys measured merely 94 feet by 21 feet, with a ceiling height of just 11 feet. Not only were conditions cramped and unsuited to learning, but the schoolmasters, Mr Harding and Mr Brown, were not averse to beating the children.[10]

If they were caught attempting to run away, the boys' heads were shaved as a punishment on their return, some were birched and others made to wear girls' clothes.[11] Children dared not confide in inspectors from their home parishes about the conditions at Drouet's for fear of being beaten. In addition, complaints of sexual assault were dismissed as lies by those running the establishment,[12] including the rape of some of the female children by Drouet's visiting half-brother, Richard,[13] a butcher from Lambeth.[14]

The Poor Law commissioners were aware of some of the ongoing abuse and made many recommendations, but these were repeatedly ignored by Drouet and his staff. The welfare of the children was of no interest to Drouet, or indeed to many others employed in so-called protective roles. The Poor Law Amendment Act of 1834 made no specific provision for the decent treatment or suitable education of poor children and gave no power to the local Poor Law Board to compel Drouet to improve conditions or even to remove him from his position. Nonetheless, the Poor Law Board of Tooting could have asked the parishes of origin to withdraw their children from Drouet's, had they believed that this would be beneficial for the children's welfare.

Moreover, some of the London Unions, or parishes, were of the mistaken belief that they could exempt themselves of the responsibility of enforcing regulations contained in the legislation. There was considerable apathy, strict adherence to the wording of the 1834 Act (where it enabled the authorities to avoid taking responsibility or incur costs) but, worst of all, even the inspectors consistently turned a blind eye to what was going on at places like Drouet's.[15] It was only as a result of events in early 1849 that the extent of the filth, overcrowding and lack of humanity began to emerge and Drouet's became known as the 'Tooting Child Farm.'[16]

In October 1848, Maria Drouet died at the family home in Margate, aged 46. The death certificate stated that she had died from 'apoplexy, not certified,'[17] the term commonly used for a stroke at the time. Bartholomew was not with her, and the informant on the death certificate was William, their son. It was later reported that Maria's death greatly affected her husband, and it is possible that Drouet's brutal behaviour intensified as a result of his wife's untimely demise.

A few weeks later, from November to December 1848 almost 90 children at Drouet's began to suffer from diarrhoea. On Friday, 15 December, three girls collapsed but Drouet dismissed their symptoms as a severe bowel complaint. Neither he nor the resident surgeon, William James Kite, took any action, despite recent newspaper reports warning of cholera and official notifications sent to all boards of guardians, parish and union medical officers.[18] On Friday, 29 December, more children began to suffer from diarrhoea and by this time, now that cholera had already broken out in London, their symptoms finally began to cause alarm. On the following night, the first child, a girl, died.[19] Yet still Drouet did not inform any of the Poor Law guardians that cholera may be present in his establishment until 3 January.

It was at this point that Dr Thomas Addison of Guy's Hospital was contacted. Educated at Edinburgh University, Addison was Chairman and President of the Westminster Medical Society, of which Dr John Snow was also a member. Although Snow's theories on the waterborne transmission of cholera would have been familiar to Addison, when he and his colleagues visited Tooting he was not initially convinced that the children were suffering from Asiatic cholera. The resident surgeon William Kite kept a note of the dead:

*31 December – three*
*1 January – three*
*2 January – seven*
*3 January – five*
*4 January – twelve*
*5 January – nineteen*
*6 January – fourteen*
*7 January – eleven*
*8 January – twenty*
*9 January – fourteen*
*10 January – ten*
*11 January – five*
*12 January – nine*
*13 January – eight*

Between 13 and 20 January there were nine more deaths, making a total of 150 fatalities at Tooting before 20 January, up to which date no inquest had been deemed necessary.[20] The final death toll, including the children who were subsequently removed to their former parishes, was 180.

An Inspector at the Board of Health, Dr Richard Dugard Grainger was the next medical professional to visit the establishment, on 5 January. Then also a Fellow of the Royal College of Surgeons, Grainger was sent to oversee an inspection and establish the cause of the outbreak. The land on which Surrey Hall was situated was punctuated with stinking, interconnecting streams and ditches serving as open sewers for the Tooting area.[21]

Grainger discovered that the boys' accommodation was built over a stagnant ditch which had once run between Tooting and Wandsworth, where there were also some cases of cholera, though it is unclear whether or not they preceded those at Drouet's. Accounts were also vague as to who had cleared out the ditches. Drouet reassured Grainger that the ditch had recently been cleared by some of the larger boys and 'men,' though it is not specified who they might have been, and Kite, the surgeon, believed the digging out had taken place under the direction of the local sanitary committee.[22] Whoever had undertaken the task, the filth contained in the ditches had been deposited on the sides, with a view to using it as fertiliser.

However, it later emerged that the clearing out of the ditch, on 6 or 7 December had been in contravention of a recommendation made to Drouet by the General Board of Health:

> ' ... *much mischief has sometimes been occasioned when the operation has been so ignorantly and unskilfully conducted ... when the contents of foul ditches have been spread out on the banks and allowed to remain there, and when cesspools have been emptied into drains or sewers having no proper fall, or no run for the discharge of the contents from beneath inhabited houses. Works of this kind should be conducted under the superintendence of a person who possesses some knowledge ... The medical*

*officer ... should ... be required to take the general*
*superintendence of such operations.'* [23]

Grainger also located a second ditch in the grounds connected to a large tank, into which drained all the refuse from the nearby Surrey Lunatic Asylum. This ditch was about 3 feet deep but some 18 to 20 feet wide and it gave off a most noxious smell. To the side of the field in which it was situated, the ditch had been dammed in order for the detritus to accumulate for use as fertiliser. In short, the two ditches were open sewers, however, the inspectors were told that the water used by the Tooting population was obtained from artesian wells supplied by an underground water source. At one of the inquests held into the deaths of the children, when asked about the quality of the drinking water, resident surgeon, W. J. Kite acknowledged that the water had an offensive smell.[24] It is highly likely that the filth in the ditches and streams on the Surrey Hall land was contaminating the water supply, and the spread of cholera was accelerated by poor hygiene and the deplorable living conditions.

Despite the evidence, Richard Grainger was not persuaded that the drinking water source was polluted by the putrid ditches. An anti-contagionist, favouring the view that cholera was transmitted by atmospheric miasmas, Grainger felt the putrid smell was of greater concern and he concluded that 'the disease arose from atmospheric poison.'[25] Yet, the outbreak was restricted to Drouet's and beyond the confines of the establishment it was evident that cholera was not spreading through the air to the immediate surrounding neighbourhood. Grainger and his anti-contagionist colleague Dr John Sutherland inspected many premises during the 1848-9 cholera outbreak, including the famously noxious bone-boiling factories to the north of Tooting in Lambeth. According to historian R. J. Morris, such inspections were 'active, powerless, derided and largely ineffective.'[26]

Grainger later explained his failure to take action at the inquest investigating the deaths at Tooting, in the following way:

'... *the General Board of Health acted under the authority*
*of two acts of Parliament. The first was the Public Health*

*Act, which gave the General Board of Health very considerable powers in all parts of England, except London, and a circle of 10 or 12 miles round the metropolis. Mr. Drouett's [sic] establishment, therefore, did not come under the operation of that act of parliament. There was another measure, the Nuisances' Prevention Act, which gave the Board very limited powers, although it conferred considerable powers with regard to the removal of nuisances, and it was under this act that the Board acted. That act, however, limited their interference to recommendations, and the institution of inquiries.'*[27]

Irrespective of how cholera and other diseases were being spread, both contagionists and anti-contagionists were at least in agreement that unhygienic living conditions for the poor were not conducive to health or longevity. The difficulty was in establishing the cause of disease, and in particular cholera, which everyone on the Board of Health believed was transmitted in foul air or miasma, including Chadwick and Southwood Smith. The belief that poor living conditions were the sole cause of disease would never prevent the outbreak of cholera. The misguided belief that cholera was spread via foul air meant that preventative measures such as quarantine were regarded as unnecessary, as explained by medical historian Erwin H. Ackerknecht:

*'The Board of Health was not the least surprised by the increased morbidity and mortality of 1848-49 as compared to 1831-32. Far from attributing it to a relaxation of quarantines, it attributed it to the increase since 1831 of those conditions which it regarded as the causes of the disease and sources of the "miasma": overcrowding, filth, dampness, faulty drainage, vicinity of graveyards, unwholesome water, and unwholesome food.'*[28]

Yet the scale of the problem, the amount of public funds required to improve conditions, and arguments about issues such as who was responsible for the cleansing of foul ditches like those at Tooting, continued to impede progress and cholera continued to spread at Drouet's. By the end of the first week of January 1849, 40 new cases had been reported, however, a statement issued by the establishment's physician W. J. Kite revealed that the situation was much graver than had been previously disclosed. There had in fact been 229 cases, of which 52 children had died and only 16 had recovered.

The General Board of Health convened a special meeting at which a decision was finally made to clear the ditches. They agreed that Grainger should visit Drouet's again as soon as possible, and on 6 January he returned with 'a gang of around 50 "navvies," in their jack boots and armed with their pickaxes and scoops.' [29] Grainger made further visits on 7 and 10 January, but the decision had already been taken by him and his Board of Health colleagues, Dr Southwood Smith and Edwin Chadwick, to remove all the healthy children to their parishes of origin, leaving the sick children at Tooting.

Little did anyone realise that many of these apparently healthy children would be carrying cholera and their removal would disseminate the disease throughout the metropolis. Omnibuses arrived at Drouet's to take the children to Kensington, Newington, St Andrew's Holborn, Wandsworth and Clapham Union, St Pancras, Chelsea, Clerkenwell, Islington, Strand, Fulham, Richmond, St George-in-the-East, Kingston, and Streatham. The 154 children who were returned to Holborn were immediately sent to the Royal Free Hospital in Gray's Inn Road. It is not clear why the children were moved to the hospital, whether it was felt they could be better cared for there or simply because it provided a ready supply of beds.

Grainger's next visit to Drouet's raised further concerns about the remaining sick children's welfare. First of all, he was shocked by the severity of the outbreak, the symptoms of which were far more violent those of the cholera victims he had previously observed in Glasgow. The 160 children he found suffering were packed four to a bed, some 6 inches apart, in small, stuffy rooms around 16 feet by 12 feet in size, and less than 8 feet high. In many of the dormitories the fireplaces had been closed; not only was there no heat but also very little ventilation. A lack of windows meant the rooms were also poorly lit. There were very few nurses looking after the children, most of whom were in considerable pain,[30] left to vomit and defecate in their beds, over each other and on the floor. There was not sufficient staff to aid and comfort the children or to clean up after them; the stench in the wards was intolerable and the sheets on the beds remained soaking wet for days on end.[31]

Despite the inspectors' recommendations that conditions must be improved, little was done by Drouet. St Pancras parish sent four additional nurses, two of whom remained for a single day, but Mary Anne Keith and Sarah Sellers bravely chose to remain.[32] They were then helped by the older boys and girls from Drouet's who had not yet succumbed to cholera or who were in the process of convalescing. More children died, and in the midst of this appalling situation Drouet's staff – W. J. Kite and his visiting medical colleagues, Mr Popham, Mr Bailey, Mr Penny and Mr Phillips – publicly declared that they were helping the suffering children and administering medicine. This was evidently not the case, but it is difficult to ascertain to what extent the visiting medical team were trying to cover their own shortcomings and to what extent they were being misled and deceived by Drouet and Kite.

Further investigations also showed that prior to the outbreak 'sufficient provision [was] ... not made for the sudden alteration of the [January] weather [of] ... the last week or ten days.'[33] The tiny playground at Drouet's was dank and wet, entirely enclosed by other buildings.[34] Here, 'the female children ... were without any covering on their heads, their arms bare, and their shoulders and necks uncovered, except the slight defence of a pinafore. A large extent of the surface is thus exposed to the cold, and congestion of the bowels and other organs must be the result.' Indeed the children's clothing did not vary whether it was summer or winter.[35] Their accommodation was not heated, despite the freezing winter temperatures, and around 150 had even been housed in a low-lying outhouse which they shared with pigs, cows, horses and poultry.

On their arrival at Drouet's, in many cases the children's own garments had been replaced with thin, inadequate clothing.[36] They were poorly nourished and unable to build up resistance to disease of any sort. Many were weak and wasted, with pot-bellies – a sure sign of malnutrition. They were covered with chilblains, sores, boils and impetigo, their eyes inflamed, wounds were slow to heal. Many suffered from headaches, ringworm and scabies.[37]

Provisions supplied to Drouet's were cheap and sub-standard, with gruel made from flour, arrowroot, salt and water. Whilst giving evidence at the inquest into the deaths at Tooting, St Pancras Poor Board director, Thomas E. Baker described the gruel as 'nothing better than bill-stickers' paste.'[38] The potatoes were often black and watery, and never given at the same time as bread, loaves of which were cut up into the smallest portions possible. [39] Boys did not have enough water to drink, as it was obtained from the girls' yard, which they were not allowed to enter. Even the girls were not able to help themselves and some would swap their limited bread ration for a drink. At mealtimes the girls ate first and often drank the entire supply of water so there was none left for the boys.[40] All meals were taken standing up,[41] and if children complained of hunger they were beaten.[42]

*The Times* reported on the Tooting scandal on 13 January 1849:

'[Food] ... *consists of meat three times a-week, pudding once, and pea-soup three times a-week. On inquiry, and questioning a considerable number of children ... the food has been defective in quality; the kind and quality of the diet also have been of objectionable character, and liable, especially in a season like the present, to have exerted an injurious influence on the system. Under these circumstances it is to be much regretted that the proprietor [Drouet] did not, in accordance with the recommendations issued by the General Board [of Health], discontinue the use of a vegetable diet. If, instead of feeding these children so often on a kind of food, pea-soup (known to exert in many cases a relaxing influence on the alimentary canal), a diet consisting more of solid and dry and farinaceous food, has been substituted for green vegetables when the cholera approached the metropolis, there are sufficient grounds for interfering that the stamina of the children*

*would have been better maintained, and that consequently*
*more resistance would have been offered to the attack of*
*the epidemic influence of cholera.'* [43]

In death the children were treated as they had been in life, with shockingly little care. W. J. Kite performed post mortems on at least seven children to satisfy himself that they had indeed died of cholera.[44] On the night of 6 January, 24 children were buried at Tooting Cemetery, and the same number on the following night. Four children were packed into each coffin. There were no relatives in attendance, in fact it was later reported that little attempt had been made to contact the families of the sick and dying, or to take into consideration the fact that many of their parents were illiterate and would be unable to read any messages sent to them at their parish workhouses.[45] Some parents were not allowed to visit their children while they still lived, prohibited by Drouet or their own workhouses, such as the Holborn Union, which refused to discharge its paupers for this purpose.[46]

There seemed to be a reluctance, even outright unwillingness, to give the pauper children any dignity in death. A General Board of Health officer, Walter Chapman, had ordered the bodies to be buried within 24 hours, allowing little time for the normal rituals reserved for the dead or for their families to mourn. Another reason for this may also have been that no money was specifically allocated for the burial of the children. James Andrews was one of those removed from Tooting to the Royal Free Hospital. He died there within a short time of arrival and his body was sent to the bone house in the vaults of Trinity Church in Gray's Inn Road. James's body was swiftly buried by gravedigger William Fillby, but then later exhumed to be examined and dissected by Dr Alfred Baring Garrod from University College Hospital.[47] The 1832 Anatomy Act permitted a surgeon to claim bodies from workhouses and prisons for dissection, if there was no money available from relatives for their burial.[48]

Within a day or so of their transfer many of the seemingly healthy children who had been removed from Tooting to Wandsworth, St Pancras, Chelsea, Newington, and Holborn began exhibiting cholera symptoms and three who had been transferred to the Royal Free died.

The number of cases continued to rise and by Sunday, 7 January four more children had died at St Pancras and five at the Royal Free.

By 10 January, the number of pauper children being buried at Tooting Cemetery was causing concern among the local population. Eighty children crammed into far fewer coffins had been interred within just two weeks. It was subsequently decided that the dead should also be removed to their parishes of origin and that burials should now take place within 12 hours. Grainger ordered that the bodies should not be 'taken thorough the metropolis, as such a procedure, if known might excite alarm in the public mind.'[49]

An inquest had been set up in the first week of the outbreak and on Friday, 11 January, when proceedings were about to resume, Drouet's absence caused some surprise and concern, as he had been given notice to attend. By this point almost 100 children under his care had perished and fatalities were also occurring amongst the nursing staff. A week later, on 16 January, an inquest began at Chelsea Workhouse into the deaths of five of the children from that parish. This time Drouet attended, and on the following day he instructed a barrister to accompany him when the original inquest reconvened. It was clear Drouet was fearful of the consequences of the accusations concerning his running of the pauper asylum. In addition, so numerous were the inquests opened to investigate the children's deaths it was impossible for him to attend every inquiry.

On Tuesday, 16 January, an inquest was begun by the St Pancras Board of Directors of the Poor into the deaths of their child paupers, in particular one boy named John Joseph Coster. The inquest also scrutinised the circumstances under which the parish of St Pancras had farmed out its pauper children. It appeared that not only was there no written contract between the parish and Drouet, but the responsibility for every aspect of the children's welfare had been handed over to him. Moreover, they had been fully aware that Drouet was making a gross profit of a shilling per week on each child.

The inquest concluded with the following statement condemning not just the actions of those involved in the maltreatment and deaths of so many pauper children, but also the system that had caused them to be living at Drouet's establishment in the first place:

*'We find that John Joseph Coster died from malignant cholera, that disease occurring in him at a time when he was suffering from the effects of an inefficient diet, deficient warmth of clothing and impure air art Surrey-hall, Tooting ... At the same time the jury most emphatically condemn the practice of farming pauper children in the houses of strangers, because the system engendered by it affords to unprincipled persons disastrous opportunities of defrauding the poor children of their proper food and clothing, in a manner the wickedness and evil consequences of which do not seem to become publicly apparent, nor to produce such adequate effect on the minds of the directors and guardians of the poor as to lead to correction of the evil until disease has produced the most awful effects on the helpless population of such establishments.'*[50]

At the inquest further evidence was supplied by the St Pancras Poor Board Director Thomas E. Baker, who had 24 years' experience of treating cholera in India. He implied that inspectors may have been bribed by Drouet: 'We did not give Mr. Drouet any notice of our visits, nor did the directors of St. Pancras take anything at Mr. Drouet's table.' Baker did not find the cholera wards poorly ventilated, and noted that the windows had been closed because of the bitter north-east wind. He added, 'Here was the secret. The windows had been closed and the children had themselves produced the poison which destroyed them. That, in my opinion, was the main cause [of the cholera outbreak].'[51]

At the inquest for the children from Holborn, the visiting physicians Popham, Bailey, Penney and Phillips publicly declared that the medical attention given to the children at Tooting had not been at fault, the children had not been badly fed, nor were they in bad health prior to the outbreak. In addition, during their investigations, the conduct of Mr Drouet evoked their 'warmest admiration [he had shown] ... kindness, humanity, and liberality [and] the utmost consideration for the children.' Their view was that any defect in the sanitation at the establishment was the responsibility of the Commissioners of Sewers.[52]

The inquest into the deaths of the children from the Holborn Union reconvened on 23 January. The inquest had been led by surgeon Thomas Wakely MP, a social reformer and founding editor of *The Lancet*. Wakely was also the coroner for Middlesex and the children from Holborn came under his jurisdiction.[53] Wakely considered who should be deemed at fault before the jury came to their verdict. He concluded that the Poor Law guardians were not at fault, 'for they paid an adequate sum for the children's maintenance, and appointed visitors to examine them, and as soon as they knew of the outbreak of disease they spared no cost to place the children in security immediately.'[54] He then considered the role of the Poor Law Commissioners, 'Mr. Drouet's establishment had not really been under their superintendence and control; they were, therefore, absolved from legal responsibility.'[55] And what of Mr Hall, the Poor Law inspector? He had 'acted under the authority of the Commissioners [and] was absolved from legal responsibility.'[56] Next, Wakely judged that the resident surgeon, W. J. Kite was not culpable, as he too had not been legally responsible. Wakely concluded that it was solely 'Mr. Drouet, the proprietor of that establishment [who] was responsible in law ... [and] ... guilty of manslaughter.'[57]

In the days that followed, the jury at the inquest in Putney was discharged, following Drouet's conviction at Holborn. However, at Chelsea, where Wakely also led proceedings, he decided that it would be wrong to terminate the inquiry, as a full and thorough investigation was still necessary. Nor had an inquest been opened for the 150 children who had died at Tooting. This time Wakely concluded that the responsibility lay at the feet of the board of guardians and Drouet, but he then backtracked, absolving the the guardians from legal responsibility, as some children had been removed from Tooting.

He did, however, observe that 'the system of farming children was an abomination. By that system they held out to persons a very strong inducement and temptation to do wrong, and to make the greatest possible profit, by giving to the children committed to their care the smallest possible amount of food.'[58] The jury returned a verdict of manslaughter against Drouet for the second time.

Within a fortnight, rumours were circulating that Drouet had died, but this was not the case, rather he had been seriously ill. Information put out by W. J. Kite implied that Drouet had a heart condition, which had been exacerbated by stress. On 9 April 1849 the trial of Bartholomew Peter Drouet for manslaughter began at the Old Bailey, London's central criminal court. He was accused of 'feloniously killing and slaying James Andrews,'[59] the child victim of cholera, who had been removed to the Royal Free. At the trial evidence was given by a considerable number of people who had visited Surrey Hall over the previous couple of years. Many children also gave evidence and the trial excited considerable public interest. The primary aim of the proceedings was to ascertain whether or not James Andrews's death from cholera had resulted from the ill-treatment he had received at the hands of Drouet.

On Friday, 13 April 1849 the trial came to a conclusion: Drouet was acquitted, and as recorded in the court proceedings for the Old Bailey:

> '... it being clear that the death being a consequent of the visitation of the cholera, and was not directly or immediately caused by any neglect of duty on the part of Mr Drouet ... No evidence had been adduced to show that the child might not have died of the cholera if that treatment had not been exhibited; and in the absence of such evidence, in his opinion, in point of law the prisoner ought to be acquitted.'[60]

The jury could not hold Drouet responsible, as no medical professional called to give evidence had been able to explain the definitive cause of cholera. Many examples were given to demonstrate how the children's underlying bad health and poor living conditions had contributed to their deaths, but no exact cause of the disease could be defined. It was therefore impossible to blame Drouet. The author Charles Dickens was fascinated by the case and reported that 'Drouet was "affected to tears" as he left the dock. It might be gratitude for his escape, or it might be grief that his occupation was put an end to.'[61]

Now a free man, Drouet retreated to his house overlooking the sea in Fort Crescent, Margate. The stress of the cholera outbreak, the public accusations and the trial had taken their toll, and Drouet died, aged 54, just a few weeks later, on 26 July 1849, of 'disease of the heart and dropsy,' oedema caused by congestive heart disease.[62] Newspapers across Britain reported his death, including the following report from the *Dundee Courier*: 'He had been nine years a resident in Tooting, and not only bore the character of a good master, but was much respected by the inhabitants.'[63] Drouet was buried at Tooting the following day.

Charles Dickens published a piece entitled, 'The Paradise at Tooting', in *The Examiner* on 20 January 1849, at the height of the crisis. In it he gave a damning assessment of Drouet's involvement in the tragedy, although he also correctly points out the culpability of the authorities:

> '... *though it cannot diminish the heavy amount of blame that rests on this sordid contractor's head* [Drouet], *there is great blame elsewhere. The parish authorities who sent these children to such a place, and, seeing them in it, left them there, and showed no resolute determination to reform it altogether, are culpable in the highest degree. The Poor-Law Inspector who visited this place, and did not, in the strongest terms, condemn it, is not less culpable. The Poor-Law Commissioners, if they had the power to issue positive orders for its better management (a point which is, however, in question), were as culpable as any of the rest.*
>
> '*The cholera, or some unusually malignant form of typhus assimilating itself to that disease, broke out in Mr Drouet's farm for children, because it was brutally conducted, vilely kept, preposterously inspected, dishonestly defended, a disgrace to a Christian community, and a stain upon a civilised land.'*[64]

It seems inconceivable that pauper children should have been treated in this way and by those whose responsibility it was to protect them. However, it is worth looking into Drouet's own background and the people with whom he was associated to understand better what was going on at Tooting and other workhouses across Britain, as the neglect which occurred here was not an isolated case.

Bartholomew Peter Drouet was born in London, around 1794, the son of William Henry Drouet and Elizabeth Oram.[65] He was probably the great grandson of the Huguenot mariner, Guillaume Drouet, who arrived in England about 1690 and settled in Spitalfields. Bartholomew Peter began his working life in 1809 at Fresh Wharf, Thames Street, London, as an employee of Mallough and Company, merchants, wharfingers and lightermen, the operators of flat-bottomed barges. A year later, Drouet's mother died and this may have prompted his apprenticeship in December 1811 to lighterman William Boak, who also worked for Mallough's. Drouet worked at Ralph's Quay between the Tower of London and Billingsgate and, after his apprenticeship, for another man called John Knill.

It is not clear why Drouet did not remain on the river, but in 1814 his father re-married and it is possible that Drouet was not happy with this new union. Drouet moved to Gosport to work for Charles Mott at the local workhouse and later to Lambeth Workhouse, where he remained for eight years.[66] Drouet married Maria Frasier at Southwark in 1827, but Hampshire records suggest that in 1822 she had already borne him a son, William.[67]

Drouet's employer at Gosport, Charles Mott, had been a shopkeeper in Lambeth during the 1820s and he had connections with the merchants who worked in the wharves at the docks. This, combined with the fact that Drouet's half brother Richard was also a tradesman in Lambeth, may have brought the men into contact with each other. Whilst the reasons for their initial meeting remains unclear, Drouet and Mott eventually went on to enjoy a formal business partnership, which was dissolved in 1834:

*'Partnership heretofore subsisting between the under-
signed, Charles Mott and Bartholomew Peter Drouet, as
Contractors for the Care and Maintenance of the Poor at
Lambeth, Surrey, or elsewhere, as Charles Mott and*

*Company, is this day dissolved by mutual consent, the said Charles Mott having retired therefrom in favour of the said Bartholomew Peter Drouet, who will alone in future conduct the concerns hereof on his own individual account.— Dated the 1st day of November 1834. Chas. Mott. B. P. Drouet.'*[68]

Mott held strong views on the management of parish finances and the amount of money that should be spent on the poor. He even gave evidence to this effect to Chadwick and Nassau prior to the Poor Law Amendment Act of 1834. In November of the same year, as a result of his evidence, Mott was appointed as an officer to the Poor Law Commission, and then served until 1842 as an Assistant Commissioner.[69] In this capacity Mott had considerable influence over how England's poor were treated and at Newington, near Lambeth, and then at Alverstoke in Gosport, Hampshire, Mott put his theories into practice 'contracting for the management of the paupers, as well or better than they were managed, and at a cheaper rate.'[66]

Mott later became the principal proprietor of Peckham House Lunatic Asylum, where he dealt with around 40 London parishes. Like Drouet at Tooting, Mott was paid a sum by each parish for every pauper he took in, and he explained to the Poor Law Commissioners how he was able to save the parishes money, mainly by cutting the cost of food. He would weigh the rations given to inmates exactly, measuring their economic rather than nutritional value. Wasted food was wasted money and for this reason Mott also procured the most competitive rates from suppliers. He also speeded up the way in which food was served to inmates, so that as it took up as little working time as possible. Edwin Chadwick and Nassau Senior, the co-authors of the 1834 Report, were clearly impressed and influenced by Mott's ideas. They also interviewed Mott's protégé, Drouet, who by 1834 had moved back to London, where he had become resident Contractor and Master of Lambeth Workhouse.

In his evidence to the Poor Law Commission, Drouet revealed that he had previously worked at Gosport for five years, and that for 18 years he 'had been accustomed to the management of large bodies of poor working men.'[70] Drouet was certainly exaggerating his experience and qualifications, as in 1811 he had only just commenced his apprenticeship with Boak. Drouet also gave a glowing report of the food and conditions at the Lambeth Workhouse. His views on the poor are revealing and his evidence suggests that he considered the poor a distinct and separate group in society, who should be disciplined and segregated according to gender. He also alluded to a group of eight girls in his care at the Lambeth Workhouse as 'incorrigible prostitutes,' who were sent to Van Diemen's Land (Tasmania) 'as an experiment.'[68]

However, it was Mott's involvement in the early 1840s at Haydock Lodge Lunatic Asylum in South Lancashire, and the scandal that later occurred there, where comparisons with Drouet become more evident. Conditions at the Lodge were as appalling as those at Surrey Hall in Tooting. Disease was rife in the filthy, overcrowded accommodation and there was strict control of the inmates' food intake. Mott was the resident superintendent and records show that he was keeping two sets of books. Just like Drouet, he was making money from the poor:

> *'The copy kept by Charles Mott ... showed a solid supper of bread and cheese with beer, but the copy kept by the steward, as a guide to issuing provisions, showed this was only issued to about eighty-five of the male patients (none of the women) who were employed during the day ... there was a uniform deficiency in the amount of milk used in the "rice milk". Fourteen, out of the forty-six quarts that should have been used, was made up of water. Even the milk that was used was only obtained by abstracting a large quantity from what should have been used in the breakfast porridge.'*[69]

Mott's contempt for the paupers in his charge and his disregard for the weakest members of society eventually caused him to lose his position as a Commissioner. Once a working class shopkeeper, Mott had become, perhaps one of the most vehement critics of his own class. As Frederich Engels would later observe, 'the bourgeoisie treats ... [the working man] as a chattel.'[70]

However, the partnership between Mott and Drouet went further and caused their shared ideas and influence to spread. In 1837 Drouet's half-brother, Alfred Charles, married Mary Ann Mott. Records suggest that she was Charles Mott's niece. In 1861 Alfred divorced Mary Ann, following her 1856 'elopement' with William Stevens. Divorce papers show that Alfred had been employed at Camberwell Workhouse and then at Grove House in Brixton Hill, the Metropolitan Industrial Reformatory School. He later went on to run the King's Head pub in Lower Norwood. Census records also reveal that in 1841 Alfred and Mary Ann were working as Master and Matron at Camberwell Workhouse.[71] In the 1860s, *The Lancet* published a series of articles on the conditions in London's workhouses and Camberwell was included. The report recommended that the infirmary and the yard should be modified or rebuilt, the care of the elderly and infirm should be reviewed, qualified medical staff should be appointed and finally that the inmates' diet should be improved.[72]

The influence of the Motts and Drouets was far-reaching. Not only did they blight the lives of thousands of paupers in workhouses across England but, as their views and prejudices influenced the Poor Law Commissioners to some extent, they adversely affected the perception and treatment of the poor in England and Wales throughout the nineteenth century.

# CHAPTER 5

# Births, Marriages and Deaths: The General Register Office and the work of William Farr

Despite the cholera outbreaks of 1831-2 and 1848-9, between 1750 and 1850, as birth rates outstripped death rates, the population of England and Wales trebled to over 18 million.[1] In England and Wales, from 1841 to 1900 the birth rate per 1,000 of the population averaged at just over 34, whereas deaths were just under 21.[2]

Studies on demographic transition have shown that populations alter in stages, and the following model is backed up by nineteenth century census data. In a pre-industrial society, birth and death rates will be similar and therefore population levels are kept in check. However, as a population becomes urbanised, an improvement in circumstances for some will lead to a decrease in the overall death rate, causing the population to grow. This rate then slows as birth rates also start to fall. Finally, the situation stabilises as birth and death rates become roughly equal again and the rate of population growth remains constant.[3]

Migration from the countryside to the towns during the Industrial Revolution caused a profound demographic shift in British society, providing the working population with steady employment, the prospect of apprenticeships for the next generation, and the possibility of improving their financial and social position. The precise reasons for the increase in birth rate at the beginning of the nineteenth century are unclear, however improvements in socio-economic status may have played a part.

Irrespective of the reasons for it, the rise in population caused by the move from an agrarian to an industrial economy was of grave concern to contemporary commentators. In his 1798 work, *An Essay on the Principle of Population*, Thomas Malthus debated whether a growing population would be able to feed itself. In the early years of the nineteenth century population growth, together with economic and political forces, put increased pressure on the ability of the diminished numbers of agricultural labourers to produce food, despite mechanisation and new farming methods.

Malthus's conclusion was that when the rate of population growth outstrips the ability to produce enough food, the population would be kept in check by 'misery and vice.'[4] Diseases such as epidemic cholera would, of course, have this effect. The British population was also kept in check by the considerable numbers of families and individuals who emigrated to America, Canada, Australia, and New Zealand in the first half of the nineteenth century. A study on migration in Britain by Colin G. Pooley and Jean Turnbull examines the movements of 16,091 people between 1750 and 1839 from information provided by family historians. Of these individuals 39.8 per cent emigrated to the USA and Canada, and 16.4 percent to Australia and New Zealand; their study also showed that some migrants returned.[5]

In addition, throughout the nineteenth century many people took up posts in British colonies across the world – in India, Africa and the Far East. Some settled permanently overseas, but many families adopted an itinerant way of life. The fluidity of Britain's migrant workforce and the economic impact of migration made it ever more important for the authorities to keep track of the population, while Enlightenment thinking and a new fascination with science also played a part. Statistics were vital in this process, which was described by philosopher Jeremy Bentham in his *Constitutional Code* as a 'Health-regarding-evidence-elicitative and recordative function.'[6]

The Industrial Revolution created fresh opportunities as well as problems, and a new urban British middle class emerged. Although wealthy, this group was unrepresented in parliament and to address this problem the 1832 Great Reform Act created 135 new parliamentary seats within industrial areas, such as Manchester, Leeds, Birmingham, Sheffield, and the metropolitan districts of London. The franchise was increased from around 400,000 to 650,000, extending the right to vote to men who owned a certain value of property, rather than land.[7] The early nineteenth century also saw a shift in mood, with the emergence of young intellectuals, businessmen and pressure groups, such as the Philosophical Radicals, who were eager for reform and with whom successive Whig administrations had some sympathy, or perhaps tolerated to a greater extent than the Tories.[8]

Government and its institutions still needed to become more representative of society as a whole. Further pressure came from Non-conformists, who felt they were disadvantaged in a society where the Church of England carried considerable economic sway as a landowner and collector of tithes. Non-conformists also had limited access to education, as in most towns in villages the only schools were off-shoots of the local Anglican church. As previously mentioned, Edinburgh University played an important role, as it produced a new breed of free-thinking, non-conformist liberals, who were prevented from attending Oxford or Cambridge which only admitted Anglicans at that time. The University of London, founded by Royal Charter in 1836, became the first university in England to admit students irrespective of their religious beliefs. Jeremy Bentham is seen as the university's spiritual founder as, although he was not directly responsible for its founding, his vision played an important role in its development.[9] Despite such moves, the Church of England still retained considerable influence in British society and perhaps most significantly when it came to births marriages and deaths, which were only recognised by the law if they were recorded in Anglican parish registers. Non-conformists needed 'a legally recognized means to prove family relationships and establish inheritances.'[10] This was fulfilled with the passage of the 1836 Civil Registration Acts.

The new system for civil registration began on 1 July 1837, coordinated by the General Register Office (GRO) at Somerset House in London and the Registrar, Thomas Henry Lister. The Registrations Acts established the new system in 619 districts, which were based on the Poor Law Unions.[11] The poor law guardians who ran each union were responsible for the appointment of a Superintendent Registrar for each civil registration district, as well as a registrar for each sub-district.[12] Births and deaths were to be registered in the district in which they took place, though the system of recording such events in parish registers continued.[13]

During the early years the registration of births was not compulsory, and today's genealogical websites warn researchers that prior to 1875 around 6 to 10 per cent of births were not registered.[14] However, local registrars had a responsibility to be aware of births and deaths within their area, to record them and then to pass on a copy of the information to their Superintendent Registrar. He would then index local records for the district every quarter, when the same information would be copied and sent to the GRO, where the entries were indexed.[15] The 1874 Births and Deaths Registration Act made registration much stricter and required, in the case of births and deaths, the parents or nearest relatives to register the birth or death within a specified period of time, and in the presence of the local registrar.[16]

The GRO was set up in 1837 during the period that Edwin Chadwick was working as secretary to the Poor Law Commission. Registrar Thomas Lister realised that someone was needed to compile statistics from the data being received and William Farr was suggested for the appointment. A medical journalist and statistician who moved in similar circles to Chadwick, Farr had already made a name for himself that year, writing a chapter in John Ramsay McCulloch's, *Statistical Account of the British Empire.*[17] Chadwick supported Farr's appointment in July 1839,[18] and within a year of joining the GRO Farr had been made Compiler of Abstracts, a post he was to hold until 1880.

The son of a Shropshire agricultural labourer, Farr had been taken under the wing of the local squire, Joseph Pryce, who sponsored his education. On Pryce's death in 1829, Farr inherited £500 to further his studies and was subsequently able to attend University College London (UCL), where he gained a Licence of the Society of Apothecaries (LSA) in 1832.[19] Following his time at UCL, where he may have originally encountered Edwin Chadwick, Farr made an unsuccessful attempt to set up a medical practice in London[20] and in the meantime supplemented his salary by writing medical articles for publications such as *The Lancet* on statistics and public health.[21] Like Chadwick, Farr was a reformer, keen to establish a link between health, mortality, population density and living conditions. He was convinced that 'disease, and especially epidemic mortality, was not only a medical but also a social phenomenon.'[22]

Farr's appointment to the GRO presented him with an opportunity to instigate change through the power of statistics. In the words of his biographer, John M. Eyler, 'Characteristically he [Farr] showed how national mortality statistics could be used to illustrate the magnitude of human suffering and premature death caused by ignorance, mismanagement, and neglect.'[23]

Lister's *First Annual Report*, produced in 1838, contained an appended letter by Farr, which read as follows:

> *'Diseases are more easily prevented than cured and the first step to their prevention is the discovery of their exciting causes. The registry will show the agency of these cases by numerical facts and measure the intensity of their influence and will collect information on the laws of vitality and the variation of these laws in the two sexes at different ages and the influence of civilisation, occupation, locality, seasons and other physical agencies whether in generating diseases and inducing death or in improving the public health.'*[24]

Farr's letters continued as attachments to his abstracts on the causes of death, which gave him the opportunity to comment on the significance of the statistics he had gleaned from death registrations.[25] The new system for the registration of deaths was of enormous value to Farr for it included not just the name, age, address and occupation of the deceased but also their cause of death. There has been some discussion amongst historians as to whether the inclusion of the cause had been Chadwick's idea, and Dr Margaret Pelling notes that, whilst it would have been consistent with his Benthamite thinking, the addition of cause of death on certificates was more likely a response to the views of the Provincial Medical and Surgical Association.[26]

Previously, one of the main difficulties of using deaths for statistical analysis had been that the cause was often not recorded properly.

Amongst various reasons for this was the fact that the cause of death was often conjecture, because many medical practitioners were not competent enough to diagnose specific symptoms and no one fully understood what caused disease. This was certainly the case with cholera, as many practitioners were not able to distinguish between severe dysentery and full-blown Asiatic cholera. In addition, doctors were reluctant to cause panic by diagnosing cholera as the cause of death in a patient. It is not surprising, therefore, that at the conclusion of the 1831-2 outbreak, the mortality figures for cholera – which were gleaned from a variety of sources, including physicians, parish records and the press – range from 32,000 to 50,000.

During the 1831-2 outbreak, prior to the Civil Registration Acts, the physician Thomas Shapter observed the practice of recording deaths in Exeter, which he regarded as unreliable. Parishioners were fearful of cholera, which they believed to be contagious, but they also fervently upheld their right to be buried in their local parish graveyard:

> *'It was also made a source of complaint that the bodies of many who had died from Cholera, were, subsequently to the opening of the Cholera Burial-grounds, interred in the common and ordinary grounds of the City, and that the certificates of the death having proceeded from Cholera, and which constituted the authority to bury in the grounds devoted to this purpose, were withheld ... the law certainly was somewhat cumbrous, and enacted but little power.'*[27]

In 1845 the GRO sent out guidance to the medical profession on how to properly certify the cause of death.[28] Medical practitioners 'were requested to accept an obligation to provide a written certificate of the cause of death in all cases attended by them which ended fatally. Deaths would thenceforth be recorded as either *Certified* or *Not Certified*.'[29] Compulsory medical certification of death was not introduced, however, until 1874.[30]

The cholera outbreak of 1848-9 provided an excellent opportunity to study rates of mortality and pinpoint the areas in which cholera was most prevalent. Yet, even when doctors were actively certifying deaths, there was still no guarantee that they were able to identify cholera symptoms correctly, and some continued to obscure the true cause of death in order to avoid widespread panic in their communities. For that reason it is impossible to know exactly how many died during that outbreak from Asiatic cholera, but the statistics were more reliable for this second outbreak than for that of 1831-2.

In addition, in the midst of the epidemic of 1848-9 it was still widely believed that the dead were contagious, and so there was often a rush, both on the part of the families and the authorities, to remove victims as quickly as possible for burial, without the proper certification. The *London Standard* reported the case of a woman in Walworth, London, who had died of cholera at the height of the 1849 outbreak:

> *'Yesterday an inquest was held before Mr. W. Carter, the coroner, at the Duke of Suffolk, Brandon-street, Walworth, respecting the death of Emma Wells, aged 44 years ... the deceased expired in great agony at nine the same day. Witness left home, and when he returned at one o'clock to dinner, he found that the body of his wife had been taken away to the dead-house, by the parish undertaker (Mr. Lane). The body was taken away in two hours after death.*
>
> *– The Coroner: Do you mean to say the body was taken away and buried without a certificate?'[31]*

Located in the borough of Southwark, on the south side of the Thames, hundreds died from cholera in Walworth and this part of London in the warm September of 1849, putting funeral directors and parish graveyards under tremendous strain. It is likely that many of these deaths went unrecorded, however in the case of Emma Wells, the local vicar was not one to cut corners, as the article goes on to explain:

> *– Mr. Cooke, the officer, here explained to the Coroner that bodies were removed to the dead-house as soon after death as possible, by orders from the Board of Health. He had*

*known some to be interred without the usual document, but*
*in the present case the clergyman had refused to bury the*
*body unless a certificate was produced.*
*– Coroner: And very proper too.'* [32]

Any friendly relationship that might have existed between Farr and Chadwick was severely strained during the initial year of Farr's appointment at the GRO and his first analysis of causes of death in England and Wales. Of the 148,000 deaths reported, Farr attributed 63 of these to 'starvation.' Chadwick viewed this a criticism of the Poor Law because, 'If people were starving, there was something about the policy that didn't work ... for Chadwick any starvation was a public embarrassment.'[33] Chadwick argued that Farr's cases involving death from starvation had been due to other causes.

Farr understood the plight of the poor and knew that starvation was occurring, but the argument highlighted the need for an accurate nosological system, that is, more precise names for the causes of death. He revised his nosology in 1842 and again in 1853, and his terminology, together with that of Geneva's Jacob-Marc d'Espiné, is still in use today in many English speaking countries.[34]

Farr had devised his first nosological table in 1837, though it was not immediately adopted by practitioners,[35] and in it he classified causes of death as follows: 'Epidemic, endemic and contagious diseases, and sporadic diseases'. These included the following categories:

*of the nervous system,*
*of the respiratory organs, of the organs of circulation,*
*of the digestive organs (intestinal canal, pancreas, liver, spleen),*
*of the urinary organs, of the organs of generation,*
*of the organs of locomotion,*
*of the integumentary system,*
*of uncertain seat,*
*old age.*

An additional cause was provided for: 'violent deaths, causes not specified'.[36]

Epidemic, endemic and contagious diseases were all *zymotic*, exuding from environmental filth and carried on the wind, then inhaled into the lungs. At this stage in his career, Farr was a firm believer in the miasmatic theory and it is therefore of no surprise that he considered cholera to be a zymotic disease.

The Public Health Act of 1848 was a milestone in the slow process of formalising and standardising a system of health care in England and Wales. Statistics were an essential part of this process and Dr John Simon, the first Medical Officer of Health for the City of London, understood this, as well as the importance of documentation and the writing of reports. Simon was a supporter of sanitary reform and he valued Farr's work. In one of his Medical Officer of Health reports for 1848-9, Simon noted:

> '*Starting then from the Registrars' Returns ... how it has come to pass that, within the City of London, there have died in the last year twice as many persons as it seems necessary that there should die; and ... here – in the very focus of civilisation, where the resources of curative medicine are greatest, and all the appliances of charitable relief most effectual ... there has passed away irrevocably during the year so undue a proportion of human life. Let it not be imagined that the word 'cholera' is a sufficient answer to these questions, or that its mention can supersede the necessity for sanitary investigation ... I would suggest ... that the presence of epidemic cholera, instead of serving to explain away the local inequalities of mortality, does in fact, only constitute a most important additional testimony to the salubrity or insalubrity of a district, and renders more evident a disparity of circumstances which was previously decided. The frightful phenomenon of a periodic pestilence belongs only to defective sanitary arrangements.*'[37]

Farr produced weekly, quarterly, annual and decennial reports, which 'helped to establish many of the standard conventions for recording and comparing mortality rates.'[38] Versions of his reports also appeared in newspapers and the publication of such information served as propaganda for those intent on improving living and sanitary conditions for the working population. During the cholera outbreak of 1848-9, newspapers such as *The Times* published Farr's reports regularly and the public was kept up to date with deaths from cholera and diarrhoea for every district of London and every area of Britain. However, the type of information contained within the reports varied. Some gave statistical comparisons between deaths and births within a specific area, others looked at how mortality rates compared to population figures taken from the 1841 Census. The reports also gave daily temperatures and included deaths from other *zymotic* diseases. At the height of the cholera outbreaks, warnings and advice were given, in addition to accounts of particularly interesting or harrowing deaths.

Farr had planned the 1841 Census with Thomas Lister with a deliberate purpose in mind. He realised that if the categories of name, age, occupation and place of habitation were all included then these could later be matched to death records, enabling him to calculate mortality rates.[39] The 1841 Census gave Farr a unique opportunity to collate and compare information. He believed disease and statistics were similar as they were both governed by sets of laws fundamental to human existence.[40]

Farr compiled statistics in the form of life tables, a technique used to measure life expectancy which he had observed in the work of the actuary and political economist Thomas Rowe Edmonds, a fellow of the Statistical Society, of which Farr had been a member since 1839. Daniel J. Friedman et al explain the workings of life tables as follows, in their research on the development of statistics in health:

> 'Farr [constructed] ... life tables from the census and registration returns: two for the entire nation, one for Healthy Districts, several for places with notably high mortality such as Liverpool and the London metropolis, and several for specialized groups such as ... British miners ... He adopted the life table as the best measure of

*the health and vitality of a population. A life table not only gave him the figures for life expectancy and age-specific mortality rates, it also allowed him to produce standardized mortality rates, typically using the nation or the Healthy Districts as standards, which allowed him to compare the mortality of places and to avoid the disturbances caused by great differences in age structure ... life tables and the law of mortality ... were the strongest proof of something that Farr fervently believed. The phenomena of life, disease and death were regular, law-abiding, and predictable, and statistics had the power to unlock their secrets.'*[41]

Statistics were used by Farr to formulate his theories on the causes of disease, in particular cholera, and to emphasise the need for widespread improvements to be made to sanitary conditions. Medical historian Dr Margaret Pelling sheds further light on Farr's methods:

*'Farr first obtained an algebraic expression for "the mean physiological duration of life in particular circumstances" based on a version of cost of living index, and then showed for London districts that their mortality rates increased in the ratio of the sixth root of their densities. This formula could ... be used to estimate the influence on a population of insanitary conditions.'*[42]

Farr's first report on cholera was published in 1852 in London. Entitled, *Report on the Mortality of Cholera in England 1848-9*, it examined deaths from diarrhoea, dysentery and cholera on a wider scale than ever before, and included London, Portsmouth, Plymouth, Bristol, Merthyr Tydfil, Wolverhampton, Liverpool, Hull and Tynemouth. The report went into considerable detail, discussing the effect on mortality from cholera by different variables – sex, age, duration, the seasons, meteorological influences, the most fatal days of the week and the fact that cholera was three times more fatal on the coast than inland.

109

The report also contained a comparison of the two epidemics in 1831-2 and 1848-9, the mortality in London during the years in which it was blighted by the plague, and a great number of tables, maps and diagrams. In addition, Farr looked at the possible causes of cholera in London, including an analysis and comparison of the following: the River Thames and the water supply; elevation; population density; and the influence of wealth and poverty.

In his discussion of the River Thames and the water supply, Farr looked at the different water companies in London and the mortality rates from cholera in 1848-9 for each area they supplied. He concluded that the highest mortality was in areas where the water source was derived from around Battersea and Hungerford Bridge. In this section he also looked at the evaporation of river water, believing that the vapours arising from the enormous surface area of the Thames were causing cholera. He noticed that there was a correlation between the higher air temperatures between May and September 1849 and increased mortality rates from cholera in the riverside areas.

Farr's observations on elevation, which he believed to be extremely important, identified that cholera was most fatal in the areas of London which lay beneath the Trinity high-water mark, in other words the low lying riverside districts. He remarked that there was a constant relation between mortality and elevation and devised mathematical equations, tables and diagrams to demonstrate the theory and confirm the relationship which he described as a law.

Farr declared from the outset that he believed population density to be of lesser importance than elevation in relation to mortality from cholera. Nevertheless, he noticed a relationship between increased density and higher mortality, but also realise that other factors were at work.

Lastly, Farr looked at the relationship between wealth and cholera deaths. He defined the worth of individuals by looking at the value of property in income tax returns. Once again Farr believed that elevation was an overriding factor, which made it impossible to establish whether mortality rates from cholera were affected by wealth. However, he remarked that wealthy people living in elevated areas were less likely to die from cholera. He concluded that those who lived in lower-lying areas, that is at sea level and on river banks, would always be more susceptible to the disease.

Farr believed this to be one of the fundamental laws that would reveal the true nature of cholera: '... it will always be the general rule that the mortality of cholera is inversely as the elevation of the people assailed above the sea level.' [43] He added for further clarification: 'The law is, that the mortality in towns of some extent and density is inversely as the elevation.' [44] Then, in conclusion, he remarked: '... the cause of cholera is some chemical modification of organic matter; and here is the great practical fact – that although elevation of habitation, with purity of air and purity of water, does not shut out the cause of cholera, it reduces its effects to insignificance.' [45]

Farr's *Report on the Mortality of Cholera in England 1848-9* was a lengthy work, and in it he also discussed the various other theories under consideration in the early 1850s about the cause of cholera, which included volcanic agency, electricity, water (and the 'practice among Native Indians of using *Boiled Water*'),[46] infection of the alimentary canal, contagion, spontaneous development and the zymotic theory. To support his elevation theory, Farr also discussed the low-lying areas in the world where other diseases were prevalent. These included ague or remittent fever in the Mediterranean and Tuscany, yellow fever in the Mississippi Delta, Gulf of Mexico, West Indies and West Africa, and the plague in Lower Egypt and the Middle East.

Whilst Farr covered a wide range of theories and ideas about the potential cause of cholera, he did not dismiss the work of Dr John Snow and the possibility that cholera might be a waterborne disease. During the 1853-4 outbreak, (discussed further in Chapter 7), Farr supplied Snow with mortality statistics which helped to support Snow's theories. Amongst the many papers he produced, Farr also wrote two further reports on cholera, in 1853-4 and 1866.

Farr's biographer John M. Eyler has written extensively on the impact of Farr's work and methods. He believes that the most striking aspect was the comprehensive and methodical nature of Farr's analysis and his firm belief that statistics would reveal an underlying law capable of explaining disease. Farr believed that mortality was influenced by the environment and statistics were a tool to help improve both: '[Farr's] approach to epidemiological research involved the use of national mortality statistics to weigh environmental influences on health, a technique of great influence in the decades before the general acceptance of the germ theory of disease.'[47]

The work conducted by William Farr did much to help eradicate the outbreaks of epidemic cholera in the nineteenth century. The introduction of the census and civil registration was an important stepping stone in the history of public health. Farr's analysis of the statistics that emerged from these records helped to cement the link between disease and living conditions, particularly the importance of effective sanitation. His methodology and attention to detail would prove invaluable during the 1866 outbreak of cholera in the East End of London. Here Farr's meticulous observations and his analysis of mortality trends helped to identify the source of contamination.

By 1866 Farr was becoming increasingly interested in the emerging field of epidemiology and Eyler notes that he was 'not content to explain zymotic diseases as the result of the introduction into the body of an undifferentiated organic material, but spoke rather of the generation, reproduction, and death of specific organic molecules, zymads or biads ... by the early 1870s [he acknowledged] the identity of independent living disease germs.'[48]

Farr's work also encouraged widespread acceptance that cholera is a waterborne disease (as will be discussed in Chapter 9).

# CHAPTER 6

# The Graveyards Overflow:
# The effect of population growth and
# cholera on traditional burial practices

In the nineteenth century, prior to industrialisation the rural and urban parish churchyards of England and Wales had ample capacity for the dead and the rituals surrounding death were an intrinsic part of life and culture. However, by the 1830s, as the population continued to grow the need for more burial capacity was becoming increasingly urgent.

Alternative cemeteries had already been set up by Non-conformists, who were unwilling to be buried in Anglican graveyards and prohibited from conducting their own services there. The first non-denominational cemetery of significant size was The Rosary in Norwich, which was licensed for burials in 1821.[1] It was followed by Chorlton Row Cemetery, Manchester in 1821; Every Street Cemetery, Ancoats, Manchester in 1824; Low Hill Cemetery, Liverpool in 1825; Westgate Hill Cemetery, Newcastle upon Tyne in 1825;[2] and Portsea Island General Cemetery in 1831.[3]

The lack of space in parish graveyards and the need for burial grounds that were open to everyone was seized upon by George Frederick Carden, a London magazine editor and barrister. Following a visit to the Père Lachaise Cemetery in Paris, Carden was inspired to create something similar in London, which he believed would provide a solution to these problems and also an unusual investment prospect. The first provisional committee of the General Cemetery Company was established in London in 1830. A year later, a public meeting was held at Exeter Hall on the Strand, 'for the establishment of a public cemetery in the neighbourhood of London, with a view to provide places of interment secure from violation, inoffensive to public health and decency and ornamental to the metropolis.'[4]

The proposed burial spaces were deemed necessary not just to accommodate a greater number of the dead – at the Exeter Hall meeting stated to be around 40,000 a year in London alone – but it was understood that the increasing number of interments within parish graveyards were compromising public health. However, there was also concern over the desecration of graves by the so-called 'body snatchers', and the supply of cadavers with which they provided the medical profession for dissection. It was not until 1832 that the Anatomy Act fully addressed this trade and legalised the use of the dead for research, when sourced from workhouses and prisons or by donation in exchange for free burial.[5]

The General Cemetery Company committee also saw the potential to create something of architectural merit in the capital, and many of the great architects of the age, including Augustus Pugin, were to become involved with the designs for the new London cemeteries.[6]

The banker, Sir John Dean Paul, who would some years later be convicted of fraud at the Old Bailey for tampering with customers' money,[7] was one of the leaders of the Exeter Hall meeting. Seated on the platform with other members of the committee, he enthusiastically showed his approval for the motion that some land to the north-west of the capital be purchased for the cemetery. He explained that, 'it was obvious that when land was purchased at £180 an acre and then sold by the foot [i.e. as a grave], the profit would be considerable.'[8] Paul clearly understood the investment potential of the project. He subsequently purchased a piece of land in London's countryside for £9,500, which was to become the first of London's municipal cemeteries, Kensal Green.[9]

The committee had also agreed at their meeting in July 1831 to 'take the proper measures for obtaining the necessary act of parliament.'[10] However, on 12 July, the day before the committee had convened in London, a vessel named the *Edward* arrived in the Humber Estuary and within a few days cases of cholera were reported in the North East. With cholera now spreading across Britain, the issues concerning the need for burial space intensified, adding to the existing high demand.

In July 1832 an act of parliament was passed to establish a 'General Cemetery Company for the Interment of the Dead in the Neighbourhood of the Metropolis.' Aware that the company's aims were not entirely for the benefit of London's poor, legislators ensured that the act contained a clause forcing the company to compensate the parishes of the deceased at a rate of between 1s 6d and 5s. Whilst the company had already sold subscriptions and shares in the scheme, they were now legitimately able to publish a prospectus and sell shares for £25 each in order to raise the £45,000 required to build the cemetery. All Souls, Kensal Green, was opened in 1833.[11]

Over the next few years, with government support, this philanthropic joint-stock company model was emulated all over the country and the following cemeteries were established:

Key Hill Cemetery, Birmingham (1834)
Newcastle General Cemetery (1834)
Sheffield General Cemetery (1836)
Fulford Cemetery, York (1836-7)
Ardwick Green Cemetery, Manchester (1837)
Manchester General Cemetery (1837)
South Metropolitan Cemetery, London (1837)
General Cemetery, Nottingham (1837-40)
Gravesend Cemetery (1838)
Highgate Cemetery, London (1839)
Arnos Vale Cemetery, Bristol (1840)
All Saints, Nunhead, London (1840)
Abney Park Cemetery, Stoke Newington, London (1840)
Brompton Cemetery, West Brompton, London (1840)
Tower Hamlets Cemetery, London (1841)
Reading Cemetery (1842)
Histon Road Cemetery, Cambridge (1843, by a private non-profit-making body)
Old Cemetery, Derby (1843)
Hull General Cemetery (1847)

Leicester General Cemetery (1849)
Overleigh Road Cemetery, Chester (1850)

The Church of England also opened some new cemeteries funded by private money, including: Abbey Cemetery, Bath (1844); Mill Road Cemetery, Cambridge (1848); and Church Cemetery, Nottingham (1856).[12]

On 14 November 1831, the Central Board of Health was established to deal with the impending threat of cholera, which was announced in the *London Gazette*:

> *'Council-Office, Whitehall, November 14, 1831.*
>
> *The Lords of His Majesty's Most Honourable Privy Council have thought fit to establish a Central Board of Health, to prepare and digest rules and regulations for the most speedy and effectual mode of guarding against the spreading of infection, and purifying any ship or house, as need may be, in any part of the United Kingdom, and to communicate the same to all magistrates, medical persons, and others His Majesty's subjects who may be desirous to be made acquainted therewith.*
>
> *The Honourable Edward. R. Stewart, Chairman.*
> *Sir William Pym, K. C. H.*
> *Lieutenant-Colonel John Marshall.*
> *Dr. Russell.*
> *Dr. Barry, K. T. S.*
> *Major R. Macdonald, Unattached half-pay.*
> *William Maclean, Secretary.*
>
> *All communications for the Central Board of Health, Whitehall, to be addressed "To the Clerk of the Council in Waiting," with the words "Central Board of Health" in the corner.'*[13]

Within a month members of the new Board, Dr William Russell and Dr David Barry, had issued an official letter outlining 'sanitary instructions for communities supposed to be actually attacked by spasmodic cholera.'[14] These were sent to medical boards across England and Wales and published in local papers. The letter included instructions such as: 'Those who die of this disease should be buried as soon as possible, wrapped in cotton or linen cloth saturated with pitch or coal tar, and be carried to the grave by the fewest possible number of persons. The funeral service to be performed in the open air.'[15]

Russell and Barry's instructions caused much consternation. They were impractical and did not allow for the burial rituals considered essential for a decent interment and in some cases, therefore, the rules were broken or bent. Many communities, including the Irish Catholic, laid their dead out at home for relatives and friends to pay their respects. Restricting the number of mourners and denying families the chance to congregate in a church for the funeral service lacked sensitivity. Moreover, the soaking of cloth in pitch or tar was not possible for most households, and the process was intolerably pungent. However, such was the fear that cholera was contagious, it was clear the deceased victims of the disease had to be handled in a different manner.

Despite the call for burying the cholera dead separately, individuals wanted and had the right to be buried within their own parish. The immediate response by local authorities and the church was the creation of new, smaller burial grounds, extensions of parish graveyards, where those who had perished from cholera could be buried nearby but still kept isolated from the rest of the community. In Upton-upon-Severn in Worcestershire, for example, cholera broke out in the spring of 1832 and persisted throughout the summer. Until the first week of August burials took place in the parish graveyard, where around 18 cholera victims were interred.[16] Fear of contagion caused the local authority and parish church to move swiftly and an area of land 10 metres by 8 metres was set aside to the west of the town in Parsons Field to accommodate the dead,[17] and here at least another 20 were buried.[18]

Similarly, in Sheffield – where around 402 would eventually die of

117

cholera in the 1831-2 outbreak – to relieve the pressure on the local parish graveyard, Sheffield benefactor, the twelfth Duke of Norfolk donated a piece of land in Norfolk Road which later became known as Monument Grounds. In 1834 building began on a design by Michael Ellison Hadfield of a spectacular obelisk to commemorate the dead, a monument that still overlooks Sheffield and has become a local landmark.[19]

In February 1832, the Cholera Prevention Act became law 'for the prevention, as far as may be possible, of the disease called the cholera, in England.' The bill required 'three members of the Privy Council, of whom one must be a senior minister, to make orders for the prevention of contagion, the relief of the sick and the burial of the dead ... anyone violating these orders could be fined from one to five pounds.' [20] The Privy Council reconstituted the Central Board of Health a couple of months later, in April. Local boards of health now had the power to 'compel local vestries to make and pay for improvements once cholera was confirmed in the area.'[21]

The responsibility for preventing and containing cholera, as well as funding these efforts, was now in the hands of local areas. In Exeter this was a problem, as works were paid for out of a general fund on which there were many other demands. This was an unusual system and different to those used by most local authorities. The statutory powers and orders that the Privy Council continued to issue throughout the summer were impossible for Exeter's local board to fulfil. Despite protestations from the city's Member of Parliament, Lewis Buck, nothing changed.[22]

The dilemma facing Exeter's Board of Health, and the terrible fear that gripped the residents of the city, were meticulously documented by the physician Thomas Shapter. A graduate of Edinburgh University, Shapter arrived in Exeter in 1832 whilst cholera was raging. In his 1832 record of this time, *The History of the Cholera in Exeter*, he devotes an entire chapter to a discussion of the local burial grounds during the epidemic. When Shapter arrived in the city two cemeteries were still in use, the Bartholomew and Southernhay, both originating from the seventeenth century, and the latter set up to alleviate overcrowding during the plague epidemics.

In the early days of the cholera outbreak these cemeteries were the only burial grounds available for victims of the disease. Graves were dug to a depth of around 6 feet and covered with a layer of lime once the plot was filled in. Shapter noted:

> *'The effect of this on passing by the burial-grounds was very startling; the white lime conspicuously pointed out the numerous deaths that had occurred, the more so as none were buried in the same grave, unless in the case of husband, wife and children ... it was subsequently ordered (Aug.2,) that the graves should be dug from eight to ten feet, and that the lime should be placed over the coffin.'* [23]

Exeter's board of health was sensitive to the views of the local population, who had become increasingly unruly. According to Shapter, there had been an incident in July while an undertaker was attending the body of a man who had died of cholera. Adhering to the rule of tarring the body within the casket, he continued with his work whilst the man's wife was suffering from the disease in the same room. The wife died before the undertaker had completed his duties and so, without wasting a moment, he ensured that her body was immediately placed in a coffin as well, and a double burial was hastily arranged.

At this time the 'underhand' method had been adopted in Exeter, as a safer and more hygienic way of carrying a coffin than on the shoulders of pall bearers. However, the combination of the rushed burial and the rejection of traditional practices incensed the crowd gathered at the Southernhay cemetery. They shouted that the couple had been 'buried alive ... like a dog', and even that they had been murdered. The unruly spectators were summoned to appear before the local magistrate and cautioned.[24]

There were further incidences of unrest in Exeter, fuelled by ignorance, fear, and perhaps even the brandy many were imbibing to ward off the cholera. So great was their concern that cholera was contagious, even the digging of the victims' graves became a problem. Shapter noted that gravediggers 'could only be kept at work by the high bribe and persuasion of frequent draughts of beer and brandy, and then when half drunk, would rarely do more than assist in digging the graves; they almost invariably refused to touch the coffins.'[25] The sextons, or officers of the church appeared to do most of the work and many of the interments took place at night.

Apart from the worry about contagion, there was additional anxiety on the part of city authorities that there would be widespread panic and potentially more unrest if the populace became aware of just how many people were dying. To that end, Shapter records that on 16 August the Exeter Board of Health asked the clergy 'that the tolling of bells in the different churches for deaths or funerals be discontinued for the present.'[26] On the whole the Church adhered to the request.

The north-west corner of Lower Bury Meadow, a field near St David's Church, had been identified by Exeter's Corporation of the Poor as a suitable site for a new burial ground. On 26 July 1832, in the belief that the new cemetery was ready for use, the order was given to bury a cholera victim there. When the local parishioners got wind of what was going on they began to 'riot' once again, according to Shapter. The unrest was such that:

> ' ... the grave-digger's webs were cut to pieces, his tools scattered abroad, he himself assaulted, and eventually obliged to fly; while the warden of the parish retained many persons in his own house during the night, in order to prevent any further attempt at the internment. It was however evident ... that this was not yet a legally constituted burial-ground and the interment of this body therein was subsequently abandoned.'[27]

By 10 August the problem still had not been resolved and a Cemetery Committee was established to settle matters. The members agreed that Little Bury Meadow was the right spot and immediately wrote to the Bishop of Exeter to ask for his permission. The Bishop gave his consent but, echoing the worry that the dead were contagious, he attached several conditions. Most were concerned with ensuring that the new ground was suitably isolated and that access to the land was secluded, so that the passage of funeral cortèges would not cause alarm to parishioners.

Three days later, the local Board of Health started to prepare the land, enclosing the area and creating an entrance off the secluded Barrack Lane (now Howell Road) and erecting temporary buildings for the housing of the clergy, hearses and for the storage of quick lime. It was agreed that those who had died most recently of cholera should be buried there straight away. In order to minimise contagion, single graves were to be dug deeper than 8 feet and double graves over 10 feet, with at least a foot between each interment. Following burial, coffins were to be covered immediately with lime.

There were still some objections to the burial ground, yet after much deliberation, on 16 August, the north-west corner of Little Bury Meadow officially became Exeter's Cholera Cemetery. The following day the local Board of Health reiterated the order that victims must be buried within 24 hours, and at the same time they reminded parishioners that this was a public cemetery and open to everyone, regardless of their faith. This caused a problem for Exeter's Jewish community, which was deeply uncomfortable that it should be forced to bury its dead in any other cemetery apart from its own. As Shapter explained, quoting a letter from the Board of Health, 'it is their universal practice, founded on a religious scruple, never to open a grave in which a body has once been interred.'[28] The Board was tested on 22 August, when a member of the Jewish community succumbed to cholera. In this case it was considered prudent to bend the rules and the victim was not buried at Little Bury Meadow.

There was additional concern that the Meadow would not be large enough to contain all of the dead. Parishioners from other parts of Exeter were also forced to bring their dead some considerable distance to bury them there, raising concerns that transporting the corpses could spread the disease. However, the authorities could find no resolution to these problems and cholera victims continued to be buried at Little Bury Meadow. Then, on 23 August, when cholera had been raging in Exeter for five weeks, a public meeting agreed that another burial ground was essential. The Board of Health identified a piece of land in Pester Lane, in the parish of St Sidwell and the process was completed far faster than for the first burial ground.

From 17 August, 159 of Exeter's cholera victims were buried at Little Bury Meadow and, from 25 August, 13 were interred at Pester Lane. Prior to this around 230 had already been buried in other graveyards within the city. Whilst the new burial grounds had somewhat alleviated the situation, the city cemeteries were still bursting at the seams.

In London the problem was even worse. In 1839 the surgeon Dr George Alfred Walker, also known as 'Graveyard Walker',[29] wrote a book entitled *Gatherings from Graveyards*, in which he included descriptions of the dilapidated and grotesque state of London's burial grounds. His accounts are graphic and gory and they make it all too evident that, even before the cholera outbreak of 1848-9, London's graveyards were not only saturated with bodies and bones, but were no longer fit for purpose. Of Whitechapel Church, Walker wrote:

> *'The vaults underneath this church, have been suffered to fall into a very dilapidated state; the smell from them, owing to the exposed and decayed state of some of the coffins is very offensive. The burial ground, adjoining the church, abuts upon one of the greatest thoroughfares in London, and is placed in the centre of a densely populated neighbourhood; its appearance altogether is extremely disgusting, and I have no doubt whatever, that the putrefactive process which is here very rapidly going on, must, in a great measure, be the cause of producing, certainly of increasing, the numerous diseases by which the lower order of the inhabitants of this parish have so frequently been visited. The ground is so densely crowded as to present one entire mass of human bones and putrefaction.'*[30]

The situation at Whitechapel was similar to that of almost all London's parish churches, but the most notorious case of all was that of Enon Chapel in St Clement's Lane, near the Strand. The chapel was made infamous thanks to the actions of the Baptist minister, W. Howse, who charged a very reasonable 15s per interment but then disposed of bodies in a most unsavoury fashion, even sending some corpses into the sewers. Walker includes a detailed description of the chapel in *Gatherings from Graveyards*, in which he reveals the extraordinary number of the dead interred there:

> *'This building ... is surrounded on all sides by houses, crowded by inhabitants, principally of the poorer class. The upper part of this building ... is separated from the lower part by a boarded floor: this is used as a burying place, and is crowded at one end, even to the top of the ceiling, with dead ... Vast numbers of bodies (... from ten to twelve thousand bodies have been deposited here, not one of which has been placed in lead.) have been placed here in pits, dug for the purpose, the uppermost of which were covered only by a few inches of earth; a sewer runs angularly across this "burying place." ... Soon after interments were made, a peculiarly long narrow black fly was observed to crawl out of many of the coffins; this insect, a product of the putrefaction of the bodies ... had the appearance of a common bug ... with wings. The children attending the Sunday School ... in which these insects were to be seen crawling and flying, in vast numbers, during the summer months, called them "body bugs," - the stench was frequently intolerable.'* [31]

Horrified by what he had witnessed in London, Walker started a pressure group, The Society for the Abolition of Burials in the Cities and Towns, to campaign for the establishment of cemeteries on out-of-town sites and the abolition of interments in towns and cities, particularly in London. The group attracted support from Edwin Chadwick, who was also concerned by the state of the burial grounds and their effect on public health.

At the time Chadwick was working for the Poor Law Commission, putting together evidence which would culminate in his 1842 work,

*Report on the Sanitary Condition of the Labouring Population.* Burials had not been included in Chadwick's report, as the issue had already been taken up by a Whig Member of Parliament, William Alexander Mackinnon, who had in 1842, as reported in *Hansard*, 'moved for a Select Committee [in the House of Commons] ... to consider the expediency of legislation in respect of interments in densely populated towns or places.'[32]

Before the Health of Towns Commission began its own enquiries, Chadwick turned his attention to the problem of urban burials and the work of Mackinnon's committee. Many witnesses were called during the 65 examinations held by the committee from March to May 1842. Dr Walker also appeared and his evidence convinced the members that measures needed to be taken.[33]

Chadwick was then commissioned by Parliament to compile a report on the findings of Mackinnon's Select Committee. *Supplementary Report on the Result of a Special Inquiry into the Practice of Interment in Towns* was published in 1843, and in it Chadwick's conclusions established a comprehensive list of the concerns over urban burials which had been discussed during the inquiry. He concluded that the stench from burials contributed to disease and therefore burial grounds should not be situated close to human habitation. Funerals could also be more appropriately conducted in peaceful cemeteries located in larger, more open spaces, while urban and chapel interments should be prohibited.

Moreover, the cost of a decent funeral was out of reach for average working people, who would also benefit from better advice on every aspect of funeral arrangement. Respectable and affordable burials should be available for all, he stressed.

Chadwick advised that the practice of keeping the dead at home for long periods before burial was unhygienic and should cease, in addition places to receive the dead, such as mortuaries, should be set up. He advised that no interment should take place without verification of death by a health officer. Once again he discussed disease prevention and the detrimental effects of the living conditions of the urban poor. His key recommendation was that sanitary reform would prolong life and therefore lower mortality rates, easing the pressure on burial sites.

Chadwick also recommended that the cost of building cemeteries should be met by loans and that a fund should be set up by parliament from burial fees, which could be put towards new burial grounds and health reforms. He also recommended that health officers should be appointed, not only to oversee every aspect of death and burial, but also to promote the importance of sanitary reform. Chadwick's prime concern, however, was to protect the bereaved poor both financially and emotionally during one of life's most testing periods.[34]

In the years that followed, successive acts of parliament were passed to improve living conditions for the working poor in Britain (as discussed in Chapter 3). A series of Nuisances Removal Acts in the 1840s gave local authorities responsibility for the health of their own area, but only when epidemic disease threatened. The acts did not create a culture of prevention in most local areas, neither did they instil in local authorities the necessity to act upon the filthiest areas of their towns and cities. The Cemetery Clauses Act of 1847 contained legislation for the establishment and the running of municipal cemeteries,[35] however, when cholera broke out again in 1848, the burial of the dead in urban graveyards had still not been prohibited.

The areas on the south bank of London's River Thames had become industrial ghettoes. Vauxhall, Lambeth and Southwark were all low-lying marshy areas where residents were packed into damp, insanitary tenements, and the river-front area between Nine Elms at Vauxhall and Waterloo Station had effectively been cut off by the building of a branch line of the London and Southampton Railway. This stretch of river was the most polluted in the capital and it was from here that two water companies, the Southwark and Vauxhall Water Company and the Lambeth Waterworks, drew their water supply (as discussed in Chapter 7). In the waterfront area there were no pumps and, as in Exeter, residents took their water directly from the river by bucket.

It was in this area that cholera first broke out in London in 1848. Dr John Snow believed that the first victim was in Horsleydown, Southwark, but it is possible that cholera had already broken out elsewhere. The disease spread swiftly and deaths peaked in the late summer of the following year, 1849.

The working poor of Lambeth still had no choice but to bury their dead in Lambeth Burial Ground, a marshy piece of land situated between the river and the railway line. On 10 September 1849, a public meeting was held at the Ship Tavern in Fore Street, Lambeth to discuss the epidemic. One of the most urgent problems was the chaotic situation at the burial ground, where a policeman was stationed at the gates to control the numbers of people entering for the 40 to 45 funerals taking place each day. By the time the outbreak was over, in the autumn of 1849, it is estimated that out of the approximate 14,500 deaths from cholera in London, over 2,000 of these had occurred in Lambeth,[36] and a large proportion of these had been interred in the local burial ground.

Dr George Alfred Walker's Society for the Abolition of Burials in the Cities and Towns continued to campaign and at a meeting of the society on 15 November 1849, the Whig Member of Parliament William Alexander Mackinnon declared, 'The present graveyard abominations must be done away with by an act of parliament. The question could no longer be delayed.'[37]

Reform had begun in the 1840s, as discussed above, and with the legislation included in the 1848 Public Health Act, which, in setting up local boards of health outside of London in England and Wales, also included provision for changes to burial practices overseen by the new General Board of Health. The 1849 Nuisances Act contained additional legislation to speed up interment, in order to prevent the spread of disease, as well as regulations pertaining to the disinfection of dead bodies and the prevention of decomposition of bodies to be used for dissection.

The first legislation to apply specifically to burials in the capital, the Metropolitan Interments Act, was passed in 1850 and began the move to end intramural interment in London parishes; the following year, the Act to Amend the Laws Concerning the Burial of the Dead started the formal process of closing London's parish graveyards. Responsibility was returned to local parishes in 1852 with the Metropolitan Interments Act, which allowed vestries to set up burial boards to oversee the establishment of new cemeteries and local mortuaries with Poor Rate money.[38]

Then from 1852 to 1857 a series of seven Burial Board Acts put in place legislation to regulate burial practice in England and Wales; the 1854 legislation gave local authorities extra powers to establish municipal cemeteries. A brief excerpt from the 1853 Burial Board Act shows how the problems of crowded burial grounds and the concerns of both the public and reformers were finally being addressed:

> 'The Public Health Act ... enables the General Board of Health ... to make public inquiry ... as to the state of the burial grounds ... After a local board of health has been established ... proceedings may be taken ... to the closing [of] any burial grounds ... [if] any burial ground ... is in such a state as to be dangerous to the health of persons living in the neighbourhood thereof, or that any church or other place of public worship ... is dangerous to the health of persons frequenting the same, by reason of the surcharged state of the vaults or graves within ... or underneath the same, and that sufficient means of interment exist within a convenient distance from such burial ground ... it shall not be lawful ... to bury ... any further corpses.'[39]

Despite the vast quantity of legislation put in place to improve burial practices, the way forward was by no means smooth. The creation of the new cemeteries would not occur without considerable problems, not least because, despite the horrors documented by Walker, the clergy and their parishioners were uncomfortable with the closure of traditional local churchyards. A letter to *The Times* published in January 1854 shows that even the most crowded parishes, such as Lambeth, continued to use their local graveyards:

> 'The parish of Lambeth is one of the largest, poorest, and most densely populated parishes in London. An order in Council was issued last year to close ... St. Mary's ... on the 31st October 1853. It appeared that [it] ... continued open, receiving a vast quantity of funerals ... kindly inform the inhabitants of Lambeth what the act really means, and

*what steps they can take to prevent their crowded parish from becoming the charnel-house for London.'* [40]

Tradition was not the only reason why local people chose to continue using old parish graveyards. The process of acquiring large tracts of land which complied with the new regulations was not straightforward. Finally, in 1854, the authorities at Lambeth were able to purchase a piece of land at Blackshaw Road, Tooting in south London and the new cemetery opened later that year. The 30-acre burial ground had cost £9,000 and less than 20 years later a further 11 acres were needed for the dead of the parish.[41] The problem of how to bury the dead rumbled on, as Britain's population continued to swell.

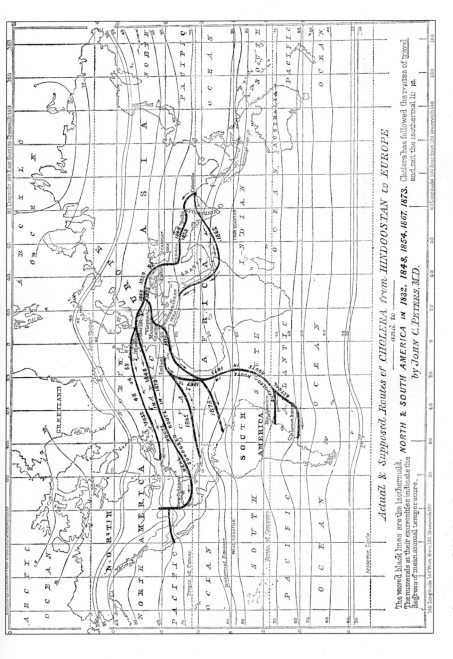

Actual and supposed routes of Cholera from Hindoostan to Europe and to North America in 1832, 1848, 1854, 1867 and 1873, published 1885; Wellcome Library, London.

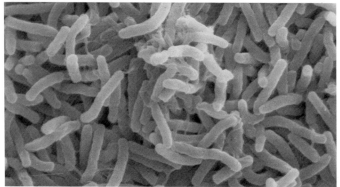

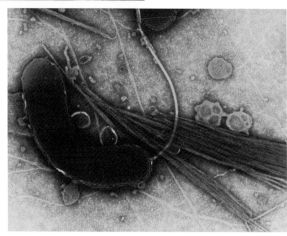

Electron microscope images of
*Vibrio cholerae* bacteria;
http://remf.dartmouth.edu/imag
es/bacteriaSEM/source/1.html

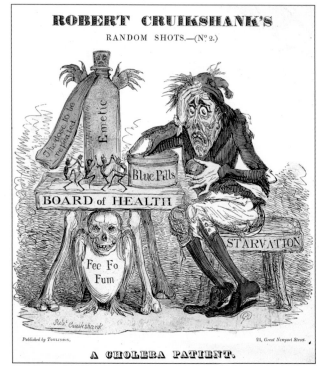

Caricature of a cholera
patient experimenting
with remedies (Robert
Cruikshank's Random
Shots No. 2), 1832;
Wellcome Library,
London.

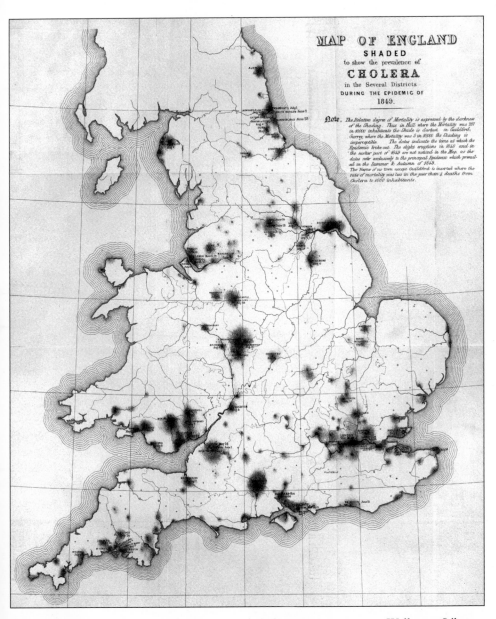

Map of England 1849 to show prevalence of cholera near waterways; Wellcome Library, London.

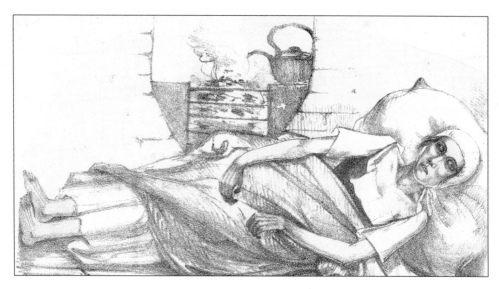

An image of a girl killed by cholera in Sunderland, November 1831, possibly Isabella Hazard (see page 38); Wellcome Library, London.

Fish Quay, Sunderland, photographed in 2013; the place where it is believed cholera first broke out in Britain in October 1831 (see page 38); photograph by the author.

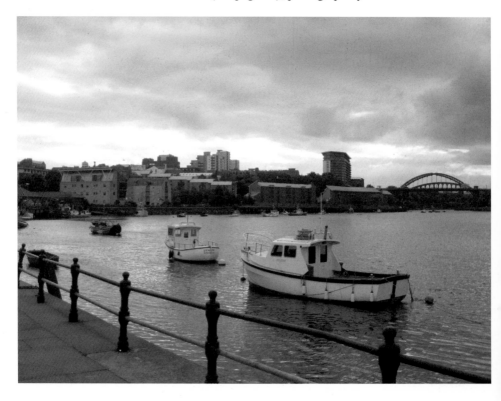

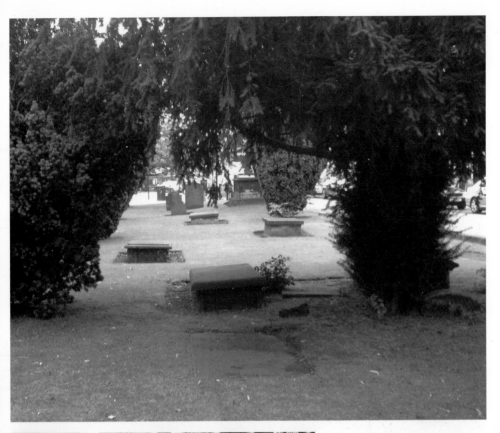

The Cholera Burial Ground in York, established during the outbreak of 1832; photograph by the author.

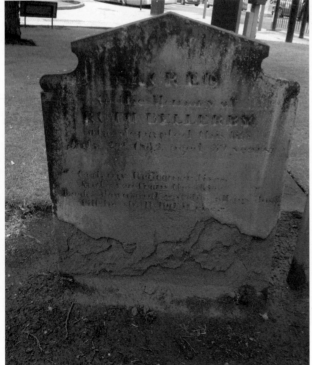

The grave of Ruth Bellerby (née Hindson) who died in the 1832 cholera outbreak, buried in York's Cholera Burial Ground (see page 54); photograph by the author.

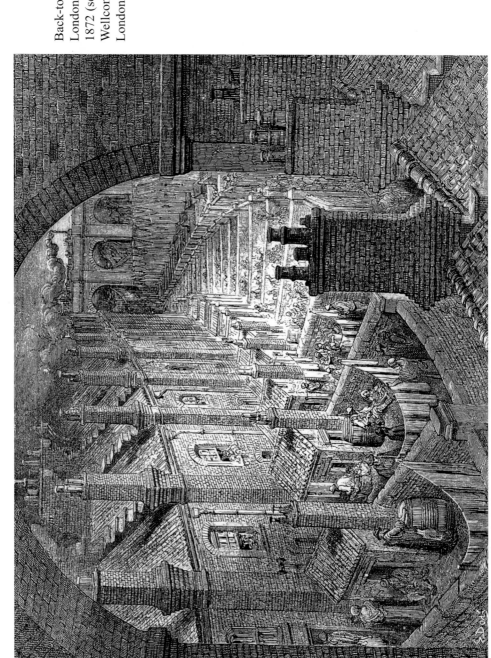

Back-to-back
London slums,
1872 (see page 63);
Wellcome Library,
London.

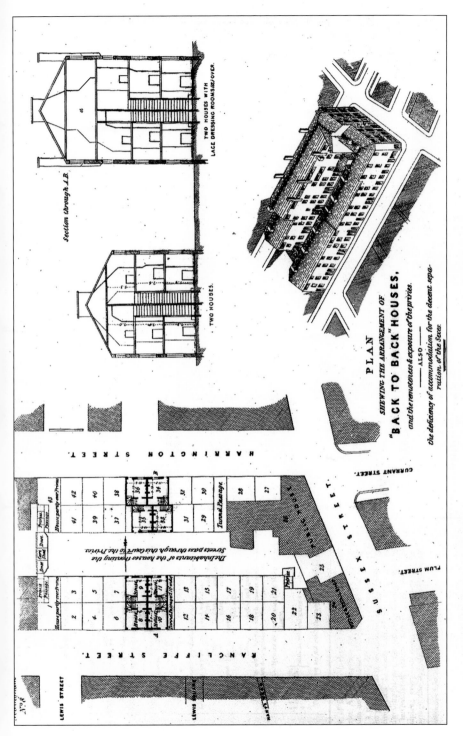

Plans of back-to-back houses in Nottingham, circa 1844 (see pages 63–4); Wellcome Library, London.

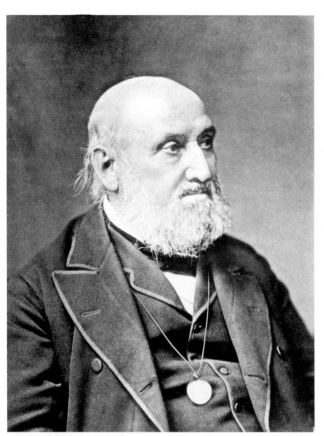

William Farr (1807-1883);
Wellcome Library, London.

Houses in London Street,
Dockhead, circa 1810, seen
from Jacob's Island,
Bermondsey, London
showing privies emptying
into the sole water supply
for the area; Wellcome
Library, London.

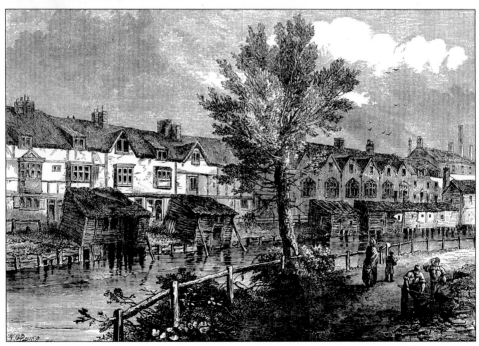

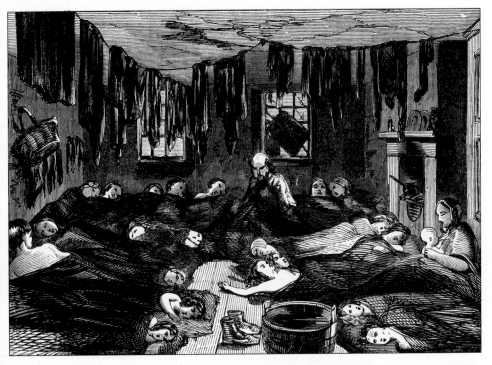

No. 7, Pheasant Court, Gray's Inn Lane, London, (Second Floor, Front Room), circa 1850; Wellcome Library, London.

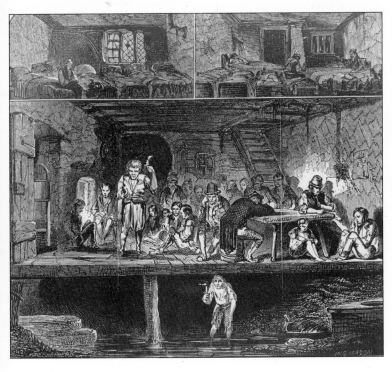

A crowded lodging house, Field Lane, London, 1848; Wellcome Library, London.

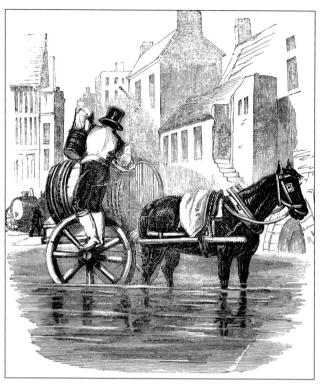

Water carriers in Exeter, from Thomas Shapter's *The History of the Cholera in Exeter in 1832*; Wellcome Library, London.

The Southernhay burial-ground from Thomas Shapter's *The History of the Cholera in Exeter in 1832*; Wellcome Library, London.

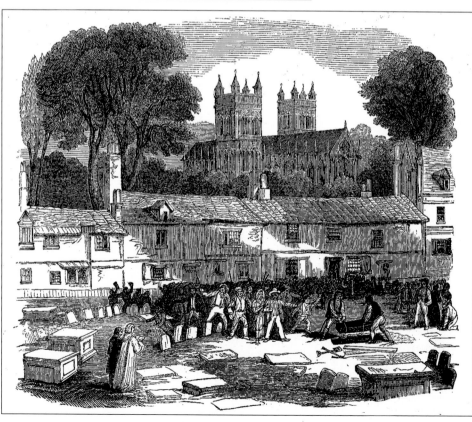

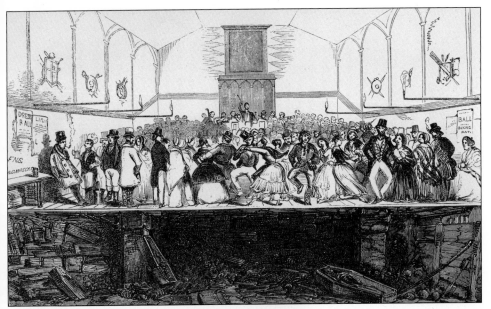

An image of the infamous Enon Chapel, St. Clement's Lane near the Strand, London (see page 122); Wellcome Library, London.

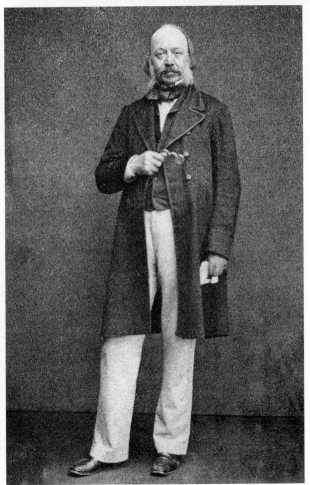

Edwin Chadwick (1800-1890); Wellcome Library, London.

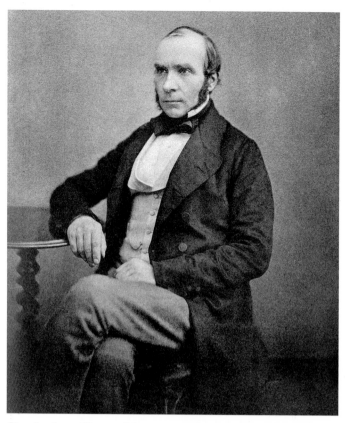

John Snow (1813-1858), photographed in 1856; Wellcome Library, London.

The death certificate of Frances Lewis, aged 5 months, who died from, 'Exhaustion after an attack of Diarrhoea four days previous to Death,' 2 September 1854, 40 Broad Street (see page 147); General Register Office.

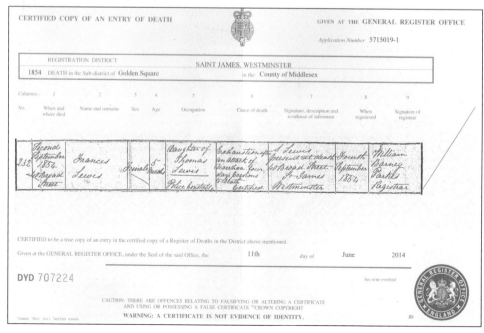

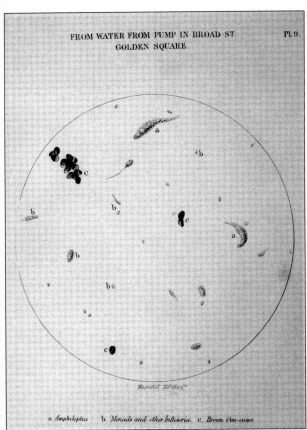

Water from the Broad Street pump, Soho, London; Wellcome Library, London.

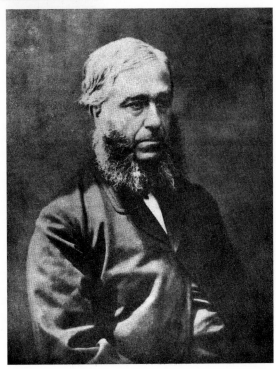

William Budd (1811-1880); Wellcome Library, London.

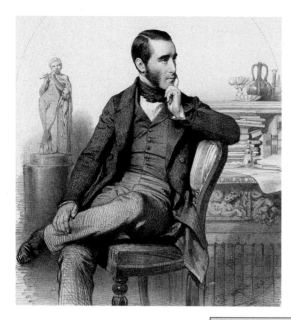

Dr. John Simon (1816-1904), knighted in 1887; Wellcome Library, London.

A slide of London sewer water taken by Dr Arthur Hill Hassall, 1850; Wellcome Library, London.

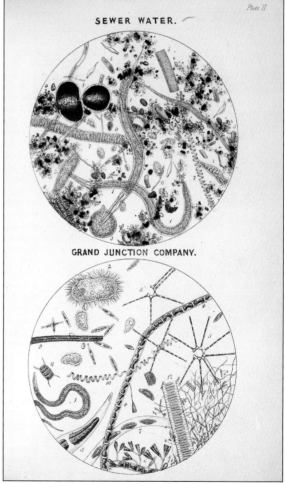

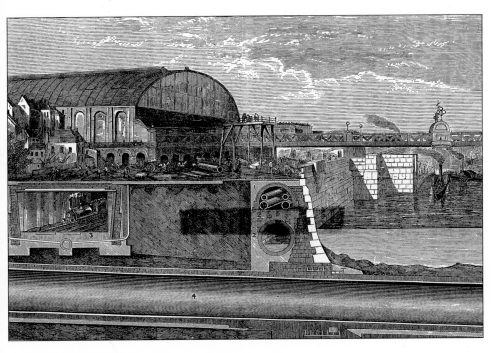

A section of Bazalgette's Victoria Embankment, 1867.
Image shows: 1. subway, 2. low-level sewer, 3. Metropolitan District Railway, 4. pneumatic railway; Wellcome Library, London.

The southern outfall works at Crossness, London; Wellcome Library, London.

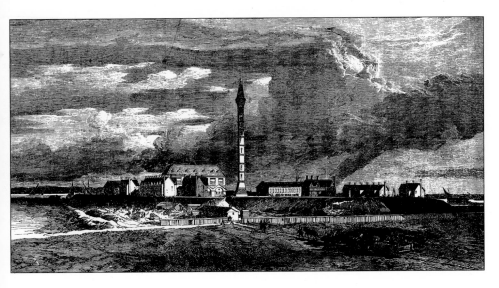

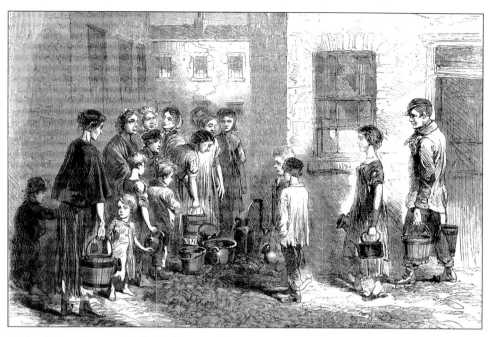

Bethnal Green's poor, 1863; Wellcome Library, London.

# CHOLERA
## AND
# WATER.
# BOARD OF WORKS
### FOR THE LIMEHOUSE DISTRICT,
**Comprising Limehouse, Ratcliff, Shadwell, and Wapping.**

The **INHABITANTS** of the District within which **CHOLERA IS PREVAILING**, are earnestly advised

# NOT TO DRINK ANY WATER
## WHICH HAS NOT
# PREVIOUSLY BEEN BOILED.

Fresh Water ought to be Boiled every Morning for the day's use, and what remains of it ought to be thrown away at night. The Water ought not to stand where any kind of dirt can get into it, and great care ought to be given to see that Water Butts and Cisterns are free from dirt.

**BY ORDER,**

## THOS. W. RATCLIFF,
#### CLERK OF THE BOARD.

*Board Offices, White Horse Street, 1st August, 1866.*

Notice issued by Limehouse Board of Works, comprising Limehouse, Ratcliff, Shadwell, and Wapping, 1866; Wellcome Library, London.

CHAPTER 7

# Dr John Snow
# and the Broad Street Pump:
# The emerging theory that cholera is a
# waterborne disease and the
# modern myth of Dr John Snow

Today Dr John Snow is credited with the discovery that cholera is a waterborne disease, but after his death his work on cholera was largely forgotten. When the new building to house the London School of Hygiene and Tropical Medicine (LSHTM) was opened in 1929, it included a frieze around the top of the outside walls. In this were carved the names of those considered to be of outstanding importance in the field of hygiene. The frieze omits Snow, and William Budd's name is also absent, yet Chadwick, Farr, Simon and Dr Edmund Parkes are all there, amongst others.

Some, including the author Tom Koch, believe Snow's fame and his reputation as a ground-breaking scientist were cemented through the writings of the early twentieth century American public health expert, William T. Sedgwick.[1] In his 1902 public health textbook, *Principles of Sanitary Science and the Public Health,* Sedgwick called Snow's work 'a monument of sanitary research.'[2] The book was used by generations of students in the United States whose study and understanding of the history of medicine was limited. In the absence of comparative examples, the myth of John Snow as the hero of cholera began. According to Koch, 'the world erroneously followed America's lead.'[3]

This is not to say that Snow's work was not important; Snow's contribution to the study of cholera and epidemiology was invaluable. His work on the 1854 cholera outbreak in Broad Street, London has been considered by many to be, in Koch's words, 'a foundational example in epidemiology, medical geography and public health.'[4]

Koch gave a lecture in 2013 at the LSHTM's 'Snow's Legacy: Epidemiology Today and Tomorrow'[5] a conference held to celebrate the bicentenary of John Snow's birth. In his talk Koch described the myth surrounding Snow as 'unstinting hero worship'; he also explained that it is necessary to 'separate the man from the myth' in order to better understand Snow's important contribution to epidemiology.[6]

Koch believes that Americans latched on to Snow because they felt he embodied the American Dream, and the Snow myth benefits from the belief that he was a poor boy who made good. It is worthwhile looking into Snow's background in greater detail to see if this really was the case. It is true that he was not from wealthy, aristocratic origins, nor was he part of the Edinburgh set, but his family were certainly not paupers.

John Snow was born in a Yorkshire village in 1813. Early documentation associated with the family records Snow's father, William, as a labourer and he probably came from a farming family in Upper Poppleton to the north-west of York. It is also interesting to note that Snow's parents had received some sort of education. William was literate, as was his wife Fanny, whom he married in 1812. Shortly after their marriage the couple moved to North Street in York, a poor area of the city on the banks of the River Ouse, which was prone to flooding. John, their eldest child, was born in 1813 and over the next few years the Snows had a further eight children[7].

Whilst the Snows clearly struggled in the early years of their married life, William's prospects swiftly improved. Between 1821 and 1823 the family moved to a house in a new terrace called Wellington Row, an extension of North Street. At this time William was working as a car man, driving a horse-drawn vehicle of some sort and probably making deliveries. However, the family's fortunes then appear to have made a distinct turn for the better. Records show that in 1824 William owned land valued at almost £38 in Upper Poppleton. Shortly after this he purchased houses and land in Queen Street, York and collected rent from other houses he owned. The money to purchase property is unlikely to have come from his work as a delivery man and the conclusion is that his change of fortune may have been the result of an inheritance. In fact by 1832 he was even able to register to vote and in 1841 he purchased a farm called Rawcliffe, where he lived out the rest of his days as a property-owning farmer.[8]

The Snows belonged to a new middle class which emerged in the early years of the nineteenth century, a group who took advantage of the new opportunities in trade and commerce in the growing towns. They understood the value of education, and for landed yeoman farmers this was not uncommon, but they did not have the funds to send their children to university.

John Snow attended elementary school in York and, aged 14, he was indentured as an apprentice to William Hardcastle, a surgeon-apothecary in Newcastle-upon-Tyne and a friend of Snow's maternal uncle Charles Empson, a traveller, book and picture dealer.[9] Empson sheds further light on Snow's background. An educated, cultured man he mixed in influential circles. About a month before Snow commenced his apprenticeship, Empson had embarked on a journey to South America with Robert Stephenson, the famous engineer who developed the steam locomotive with his father George, and who is considered one of the most important figures of the industrial age. In October 1849 Robert Stephenson became Member of Parliament for Whitby, and with other eminent engineers of the day, he also worked on the third Metropolitan Commission of Sewers in London. The Stephensons were from Killingworth near Newcastle and William Hardcastle, to whom Snow was apprenticed, was their family doctor.[10]

During his time with Hardcastle, Snow enrolled in a new medical school in York and visited Newcastle Infirmary, where the senior surgeon was Thomas Michael Greenhow, a graduate of Edinburgh University.[11] Greenhow clearly influenced the young Snow. He had an excellent reputation and understood the importance of cleanliness at a time when the value of good hygiene was little regarded. He was also deeply concerned with the plight of the poor in Newcastle and, following the 1832 cholera epidemic, wrote of his fears that the disease

131

would return should the city authorities ignore the problems of overcrowding, dirt, poor sanitation and bad air.[12]

Hardcastle worked under Greenhow at the Newcastle Lying-in Hospital, but Hardcastle was also the doctor for the coal mines at Killingworth. In 1832, as the cholera epidemic continued to rage, Hardcastle was appointed as a Poor Law Medical Officer to the parish of St John's in Newcastle and he sent Snow to Killingworth as an unsupervised assistant.[13] The experience at Killingworth was one that remained with Snow and on which he would draw in later life. He described the manner in which cholera spread in the mines within his 1855 work, the second edition of *On the Mode of Communication of Cholera*:

> *'The mining population of Great Britain have suffered more from cholera than persons in any other occupation – a circumstance which I believe can only be explained by the mode of communication of the malady above pointed out. Pitmen are differently situated from every other class of workmen in many important particulars. There are no privies in the coal pits, or, as I believe, in other mines. The workmen stay so long in the mines that they are obliged to take a supply of food with them, which they eat invariably with unwashed hands, and without knife and fork.*
>
> *'... the women and children who do not work in the mines, were attacked in as large numbers as the men. I believe, however, that this is only what ought to occur from the propagation of the cholera in the crowded dwellings of the pitmen, in the manner previously explained. The only effect of its communication in the pits would be, that the men and boys in a family would have the cholera a day or two earlier than the women and children; and if a special inquiry were made on this point, this would probably be found to be the case. It has often been said that, if cholera were a communicable disease, women ought to suffer in much greater numbers than the men, as they are employed in nursing the sick.'*[14]

In 1833, his apprenticeship at an end, Snow became assistant to the general practitioner John Watson in Burnopfield, a town south of Newcastle. A year later he took an assistantship with Joseph Warburton, a general practitioner in Pateley Bridge, North Yorkshire. The time he spent in Yorkshire helped to form some of Snow's ideas about the way in which epidemic diseases are transmitted. One of his many observations was that underground workers such as miners who were deprived of daylight appeared to suffer from worse health.[15] As with his work later in London's Soho, Snow based his conclusions on intelligent observation. Yet it is only very recently that scientists have begun to fully appreciate the essential role vitamin D plays in the human immune system.

It was during this period that Snow became interested in vegetarianism. He was profoundly influenced by the ideas of Dr William Lambe, a Fellow of the Royal College of Physicians, who emphasised the correlation between poor health and limited nutrition.[16] Lambe's philosophy influenced the way in which Snow conducted his own life and reinforced his belief that good food and clean water were essential for good health.

During his time at Pateley Bridge, Snow also came under the influence of the Temperance Movement, which was beginning to gain support in the 1820s, and he took the pledge to abstain from alcohol.[17] Together with a teacher named William Laycock, Snow organised what would later become the York Temperance Society. Snow became an enthusiastic advocate of his new vegetarian, teetotal regime, which began to intertwine with his ideas on medicine and his belief in the healing power of nature. At this time alcohol was a daily part of most people's lives and brandy was often used as a medicine. Snow, however, felt that alcohol was harmful in every respect:

> 'Nurses, and people who go about the sick, make it an excuse for taking these liquors that they keep away infection; but that is so far from being the case, that the use of them not only makes people more liable to fevers, and, indeed, most complaints, but leaves them much less chance of recovery.'[18]

133

Yet the alternative to alcohol for most people, was water, and accessing a pure water supply, particularly in more densely populated areas, was becoming more difficult.

In 1836 Snow moved to London, but in order to practise as a surgeon and apothecary he had to fulfil the educational requirements of the Royal College of Surgeons and the Society of Apothecaries. Snow took lodgings at 11 Bateman's buildings, off Soho Square, which began his long association with an interest in the area, and in October he joined the Hunterian School of Medicine in Great Windmill Street, Soho. The Hunterian School of Medicine had been set up by William Hunter and his brother John, both Edinburgh University graduates.[19] The facilities at the school were considerably better than others, as the Windmill Street premises had been designed specifically, and the fees were also good value.[20]

During his time at the Hunterian School, Snow enrolled at Westminster Hospital where he gained experience in surgical procedures. He also developed his already keen observational skills, which would undoubtedly prove useful in the years to come, both in his work on gases and cholera.[21] In May 1838 Snow passed the examination to be admitted as a member of the Royal College of Surgeons, although he had to wait until October to take the examinations for the Society of Apothecaries.[22]

Snow did not have an easy path – he did not enjoy a privileged education, nor was he part of the elite group of graduates from Edinburgh or University College London. Nevertheless, he gained his MD from the University of London, became a licentiate of the Royal College of Physicians and, as a result of his ground-breaking work on gases, was held in such great regard as an anaesthetist that he was selected to administer chloroform to Queen Victoria during childbirth.

In October 1838, Snow moved to 54 Frith Street in Soho and established his surgery in one of London's most densely populated areas. There were plenty of people to help, but he also had to compete with many other medical practitioners nearby. Snow became surgeon to four friendly societies, treating working people who had paid into a fund for medical care.

As Snow was a licentiate, rather than a fellow of the Royal College of Physicians, and had also not been taken under the wing of one of the better known London surgeons, he was never to become a physician in upper class circles, though this may have been his preference. He was highly respected in Soho, a font of advice for his colleagues and also extremely competent at midwifery. It is interesting to note that later when he could have become a fellow of the Royal College of Surgeons, he chose not to do so, preferring to work in Soho treating those who were in greater need.[23]

In 1843 Snow was elected as a fellow of the Royal Medical and Chirurgical Society, though he appeared to have a greater enthusiasm for the Westminster Medical Society which he had joined while he was still a student. Westminster was less traditional and there he could debate fresh ideas. Snow was part of a new breed of medical men, basing his theories on observation but also employing ideas from chemistry, anatomy and physics.[24] Today this would not be considered out of the ordinary for someone in medicine, but in the nineteenth century, the approach was ground-breaking.

Snow's membership of the Westminster Medical Society was to be a turning point in his career. At a meeting in the summer of 1848 the surgeon, Francis Hird, read a paper entitled, 'The Pathology and Treatment of Cholera'. Snow disagreed with Hird's view that cholera was a form of asphyxia and that sufferers benefited from the application of heat to their bodies.[25] By now cholera had broken out in Britain once again, and in London there were already cases on the southern banks of the Thames. Snow was observing the disease's progress and using his experience at Killingworth as a comparison.

Within a year, Snow had published *On the Mode of Communication of Cholera*, a treatise on cholera and its transmission. It set out his theory that cholera is transmitted by humans and new infections are seeded by individuals arriving from places where the disease is already prevalent. He considered the miasmatist view that cholera is spread through the air, poisoning the blood by inhalation. However, his conclusion was that infection was localised to the alimentary canal and caused by water tainted with contaminated sewage.

Snow had been observing the behaviour and living conditions of people in Southwark and Lambeth, and in the 1849 paper he discussed in great detail examples from Horsleydown in Southwark and Albion Terrace on Wandsworth Road. Following the publication of the paper, Snow continued working on his theories, sharing his ideas with colleagues and looking at further evidence, such as reports by parliamentary committees and case reports by other surgeons.[26]

A few weeks later, on 13 October 1849, and as the second great cholera epidemic in London was on the wane, Snow delivered another paper to the Westminster Medical Society, entitled, 'On the Pathology and Mode of Communication of Cholera'. The paper, which was later published in the *London Medical Gazette,* included a considerable amount of additional evidence and was more detailed than his earlier work. In it Snow rejects the miasmatist stance and affirms his belief that cholera infects the alimentary canal, ingested by swallowing contaminated water. His extensive work on gases and the function of the lungs may have convinced him that cholera could not be contracted through inhalation, although recent work on Crohn's disease (as discussed in Chapter 1) may eventually prove this theory to be flawed.

However, Snow was persuaded by the mounting weight of evidence suggesting that cholera might be waterborne. He noticed that cholera was worst in areas where the main source of drinking water was from filthy, sewage-infested rivers like the Thames, and that outbreaks were isolated and confined to those areas. If cholera could spread through the air, as the miasmatists believed, then it would always spread much farther afield.[27]

Snow belonged to various organisations, including the Royal Medical and Chirurgical Society, and the group that would eventually become the British Medical Association (BMA), the Provincial Medical and Surgical Association. Such affiliations were essential for debate and the dissemination of Snow's theories on cholera, including his conviction that cholera could not be transmitted through the air. Snow and the surgeon J. H. Tucker also founded a new organisation, the Epidemiological Society of London, in July 1850.[28] Five years later, the society was so well established that it began publishing its own journal, the *Journal of Public Health and Sanitary Review*, which promoted the discussion of disease.

Throughout the 1840s and 50s, Snow wrote prolifically on gases and the use of chloroform, as well as on cholera and sanitation. By the summer of 1851, his theories on cholera were becoming more fine-tuned, but his reports were often published in haste and had to be amended with subsequent editions. A further paper, characteristically presented in two parts to the Epidemiological Society in 1851, was entitled 'On the Mode of Propagation of Cholera'. This paper outlined his research even more extensively than before, with many more examples and statistics and an emphasis on the prevention of cholera through the adoption of better sanitation.[29] During this period, Snow also realised that the mortality statistics compiled by William Farr at the General Register Office were of vital importance in revealing how cholera was spread.

Snow came to the conclusion that the cause of cholera should be considered in three different ways. First, infection could occur by isolated and close contact with victims, and through the washing of tainted materials. Second, it could be caught from a single infected source, such as a contaminated well. Third, the population could be infected on a large scale from multiple sources, such as municipal water supplies.[30] His waterborne theory, whereby cholera could only infect by oral ingestion, was still considered inexact and unsubstantiated, and encountered much opposition. Snow had still not won over the miasmatists or overcome the alternative arguments of his opponents. Indeed, this was one of Snow's core problems. For whatever reasons, London's medical elite did not accept him or his theories, and Snow did not manage to win them over. In the words of Tom Koch, 'Science is never about being right, it is about convincing others that you are right.'[31]

In 1852 Snow moved to 18 Sackville Street on the other side of Regent Street, between Burlington Gardens and Piccadilly. The move to Sackville Street coincided with a twist of fate that was to provide Snow with an opportunity to help prove his cholera theory. In the same year, the Metropolis Water Act began the process that would compel London's water companies to draw their supplies from further up river. The new rules were to come into effect from 1857, by which time no water was to be taken from the Thames lower than Teddington Lock.'[32]

During the 1848-9 cholera outbreak some of the highest mortality rates in the country were located in London's south bank areas of Lambeth and Southwark. These districts were supplied by the Lambeth Waterworks and the Southwark and Vauxhall Water Company, which took their supplies from one of the most polluted stretches of the river around Battersea and Hungerford Bridge. It should also be recognised that such was the poverty within these communities that most of the waterfront population took their water directly from the Thames in buckets. In response to the 1852 Metropolis Water Act, the Lambeth Waterworks moved up river to Thames Ditton, a scheme undertaken for the company by the engineer James Simpson who installed sand filter beds at the new facility.[33]

When cholera broke out again in 1853, Snow used Farr's mortality statistics to show how death rates differed between the areas supplied by the Lambeth Waterworks or the Southwark and Vauxhall companies. In early January 1855 these were published in his *On the Mode of Communication of Cholera*. In this excerpt Snow explains the difference between the water supply of the two South London companies and the difficulty of ascertaining which water inhabitants were drinking. He also discusses his collaboration with Farr and how statistics had played a key role in determining his waterborne theory:

'The Lambeth Company removed their water works, in 1852, from opposite Hungerford Market to Thames Ditton; thus obtaining a supply of water quite free from the sewage of London. The districts supplied by the Lambeth Company are, however, also supplied, to a certain extent, by the Southwark and Vauxhall Company, the pipes of both companies going down every street, in the places where the supply is mixed, as was previously stated. In consequence of this intermixing of the water supply, the effect of the alteration made by the Lambeth Company on the progress of cholera was not so evident, to a cursory observer, as it would otherwise have been. It attracted the attention, however, of the Registrar-General, who published a table in the "Weekly Return of Births and Deaths" for 26th November 1853 ... It thus appears that *the districts partially supplied with the improved water suffered much less than the others, although, in 1849, when the Lambeth Company obtained their supply opposite Hungerford Market, these same districts suffered quite as much as those supplied entirely by the Southwark and Vauxhall Company.'* [34]

The 1855 edition of *On the Mode of Communication of Cholera* was the culmination of Snow's research and theories up to that point in his career, and it includes the story of the Broad Street water pump. Situated in London's Soho, Broad Street was an area Snow knew very well, and the violent outbreak of cholera there in August 1854 was to provide him with a hands-on opportunity for research:

*'The most terrible outbreak of cholera which ever occurred in this kingdom, is probably that which took place in Broad Street, Golden Square, and the adjoining streets, a few weeks ago. Within two hundred and fifty yards of the spot where Cambridge Street joins Broad Street, there were upwards of five hundred fatal attacks of cholera in ten days. The mortality in this limited area probably equals any that was ever caused in this country, even by the plague; and it was much more sudden, as the greater number of cases terminated in a few hours. The mortality would undoubtedly have been much greater had it not been for the flight of the population ... in less than six days from the commencement of the outbreak, the most afflicted streets were deserted by more than three-quarters of their inhabitants.'* [35]

Contrary to much that has been written on the subject, Snow's work in Soho was not conducted alone. He gleaned information from other local physicians and employed the help of the Reverend Henry Whitehead, the Curate of St Luke's Church in nearby Berwick Street, who conducted most of the door-to-door enquiries on Snow's behalf.[36]

Broad Street is situated in the Parish of St James, Westminster. In 1854 it occupied an area of 164 statute acres and the population, according to the 1851 Census, was 36,406. The parish was divided into three sub-districts: St James's Square, Golden Square, and Berwick Street. It is surrounded by Mayfair and Hanover Square (St George's) to the west; All-Souls, Marylebone, to the north; St Anne's, Soho, to the east; and Charing Cross (St Martin's-in-the-Fields) to the south.[37] Today, all of these districts are part of the City of Westminster and Broad Street is known as Broadwick Street.

St James's had not been badly affected by the cholera outbreaks of 1831-2 or 1848-9, but things would be different in 1853, when cholera struck again in London, during a warm July. In accordance with his belief that cholera had been transported to Britain from abroad, and was not caused by an endemic strain, on 12 August 1854 Snow wrote a letter to the *Medical Times and Gazette*:

> 'The following occurs in the last return of the Registrar-General:
>
> "In the same sub-district (St. James, Bermondsey,) at 10, Marine-street, on 24th July, a mate-mariner, aged 34 years, 'Asiatic cholera (101 hours,) after premonitory diarrhoea (16½ hours.).' The medical attendant states: 'This patient was chief-mate to a steam-vessel taking stores to and bringing home invalids from the Baltic fleet. Three weeks ago he brought home in his cabin the soiled linen of an officer who had been ill. The linen was washed at his house and returned."
>
> 'This was not one of the first cases, and therefore I do not quote it as actually introducing the cholera into London, but only to show the kind of intercourse that has been going on between the Baltic and the Thames. It is probable that a few simple regulations respecting this intercourse might have kept London free from the cholera, and inflicted no hardship on anybody; but, unfortunately, the chief advisers of Government in sanitary matters have had their minds occupied about drain-pipes and bad smells, and have neglected the specialities connected with the propagation of individual diseases.'[38]

Deaths continued until October 1853 and then, just as in 1848, as the weather cooled the number of deaths began to fall significantly. Deaths from diarrhoea continued throughout the entire period and then increased once more the following July, peaking between 1 and 3 September. By the end of the first week of September, over 2,000 victims had succumbed to the disease in London, before a decline in October. Of a population of just over two and a half million in London, the epidemic of 1853-4 claimed around 17,000 lives.[39]

On 23 September 1854, in another article published in the *Medical Times and Gazette*, Snow explained how he had consulted the official mortality statistics at the GRO for the sub districts of Golden Square, Berwick Street and St Ann's in Soho, for the week ending 2 September 1854.[40] Snow noted that in the first week of the outbreak, up to 2 September, 89 deaths had been registered in the Golden Square area: six from Sunday, 27 August to Wednesday, 30 August; four on Thursday, 31 August; and then 79 on Friday, 1 September and Saturday, 2 September. Thursday, therefore, marked the beginning of the outbreak.

He elaborated on this in the 1855 edition of *On the Mode of Communication of Cholera*:

> *'The irruption* [sic] *was extremely sudden, as I learn from the medical men living in the midst of the district, and commenced in the night between the 31st August and 1st September. There was hardly any premonitory diarrhoea in the cases which occurred during the first three days of the outbreak; and I have been informed by several medical men, that very few of the cases which they attended on those days ended in recovery.'*[41]

From Whitehead's door-to-door investigations and his own knowledge of the area, Snow deduced that all the victims of the outbreak had lived within a short walking distance of the water pump in Broad Street. Relatives of the dead confirmed the pump as the source of their drinking water, moreover it was known to have the water with the best taste and appearance.

Snow also noted that in three other cases the dead were children who had attended a school close to the pump. The remaining two deaths were outside the area, yet within walking distance of the Broad Street pump and therefore part of the wider epidemic. It would not have been helpful at this stage for Snow to have mentioned that cholera was prevalent elsewhere in the capital, as this would have certainly fuelled the miasmatist debate. Snow calculated that 61 of those who had died from cholera in the Broad Street area had lived within walking distance of the pump and had drunk from it, in his words, 'either constantly or occasionally,'[42] while just six of the deceased had not.

Snow realised that the mortality rate was probably even greater and more widespread. He explained that many people would not even have been aware that they had drunk other beverages which had been made with water drawn from the pump:

> '... it must be obvious that there are various ways in which the deceased persons may have taken it without ... knowledge .... The water was used for mixing with spirits in all the public houses ... dining-rooms and coffee-shops. The keeper of a coffee-shop in the neighbourhood, which was frequented by mechanics, and where the pump-water was supplied at dinner time, informed me (on 6th September) that she was already aware of nine of her customers who were dead. The pump-water was also sold in various little shops, with a teaspoonful of effervescing powder in it, under the name of sherbet; and it may have been distributed in various other ways with which I am unacquainted. The pump was frequented much more than is usual, even for a London pump in a populous neighbourhood.'[43]

In the face of potentially fierce opposition from the miasmatists, Snow included further evidence to cement his theory that cholera was not spreading through the air. He noted that although the workhouse in Poland Street was within walking distance of the pump in Broad

Street, and 'is more than three-fourths surrounded by houses in which deaths from cholera occurred ... out of five hundred and thirty-five inmates only five died of cholera;'[44] the inmates had their own supply of water.

Snow also noted that at the brewery in Broad Street, situated at the heart of the outbreak, of the 70 men employed there, whilst a couple were mildly affected, not one had died from cholera. The brewery did not use the pump water, as there was a deep well on the premises, yet at the percussion cap factory nearby, two tubs of Broad Street pump water were kept for the workers' consumption and here 18 had died of cholera.

Snow's enquiries included conversations with Dr Peter Marshall, a surgeon from Greek Street in Soho. Marshall described the case of a family in nearby Berwick Street, who had drunk from the Broad Street pump on the Sunday and then travelled to Gravesend in Kent. The mother had died just over a week later, having also, no doubt, further tainted the waters of the Thames Estuary on which Gravesend is situated. Another surgeon, Dr Fraser of Oakley Square, described the case of:

> '... a gentleman in delicate health [who] was sent for from Brighton to see his brother at 6 Poland Street ... was attacked with cholera and died in twelve hours, on 1 September. The gentleman arrived after his brother's death, and did not see the body. He only stayed about twenty minutes in the house, where he took a hasty and scanty luncheon of rumpsteak, taking with it a small tumbler of brandy and water, the water being from Broad Street pump.'[45]

The man died the following evening; clearly the addition of brandy in his water had not helped.

Fraser also communicated the most well-known story of all, that of the lady at Hampstead, which Snow felt was 'perhaps the most conclusive of all in proving the connection between the Broad Street pump and the outbreak of cholera.'[46] The woman was the widow of a percussion cap maker and, as she had once lived in the Broad Street area, she was fond of the water from the Broad Street pump. Her son had told Fraser how a cart regularly travelled from the Broad Street factory to Hampstead which customarily carried a large bottle of water for her from the pump. She received a delivery on Thursday, 31 August, and she and her niece drank from the bottle during the following days. The widow became ill on the Friday evening and died from cholera on the Saturday, swiftly followed by her niece, who died after returning to her own home 'in a high and healthy part'[47] of Islington.

Whether or not this was a reference to Farr's theories that cholera was less common in areas of elevated habitation, Snow understood the relevance and importance of Fraser's story. Snow noted that there was no cholera at this time in Hampstead or Islington, and the only possible conclusion could be that the disease had been transmitted in the bottle of water from the Broad Street pump. Later, in a letter of 23 September to the *Medical Times and Gazette*, Snow explained how he 'suspected some contamination of the water of the much frequented street-pump in Broad-street.'[48]

In the midst of the outbreak, on 3 September Snow visited the pump to inspect the quality of the water. He could see nothing to indicate that the water was tainted, but continued to monitor it over the next couple of days. He realised the quality of the water varied which, in his opinion, accounted for the rise and fall of the outbreak and noted: 'on close inspection, in the form of small white, flocculent particles; and I concluded that, at the commencement of the outbreak, it might possibly have been still more impure.'[49]

Snow later confirmed that the death toll from cholera in the Broad Street area over the days of 1 and 2 September was at least 197. His investigations had convinced him that the cholera must have originated from a single source, as the outbreak in Soho had been so violent and mortality rates were much higher than the surrounding area. If this source was the pump in Broad Street, then he might also be able to prove that cholera was a waterborne disease. What Snow did next earned him a place in history: 'I had an interview with the Board of Guardians of St. James's parish, on the evening of the 7th inst., and represented the above circumstances to them. In consequence of what I said, the handle of the pump was removed on the following day.'[50]

Despite Snow's heroic efforts in persuading the guardians to remove the pump handle, deaths from cholera had already started to decrease, either because the disease was already on the wane or because many people had left the area. It is debatable whether its removal made a real difference.

Following the outbreak, further investigations were carried out by the General Board of Health and the Commission of Sewers. Then, on 23 November 1854, the vestry of the parish of St James also set up a committee. This was eventually to include Dr Edwin Lankester (who had instigated the process), Messrs F. Crane and T. H. Rice (the two Churchwardens), Henry Bidgood, Joseph Brown, William Geesin, Charles Harrison and Thomas Watkins; later additions included the Reverend Thomas Beames, J. G. French, John James, Dr Richard King, John Marshall, G. W. Sanford, Rev. Henry Whitehead and Dr John Snow.

It was likely through the committee that Snow first met Whitehead, who would subsequently assist him with his research and door-to-door enquiries. Lankester had originally intended to restrict the committee to only eight members, but the General Board of Health refused to allow him to use their reports on the outbreak, as it was felt the inquiry should be conducted in an independent manner. As a result, Lankester needed more people to be involved, which was to prove fortuitous.[51]

Prior to writing his report for the committee, Snow produced some material to illustrate his hypothesis on the cause of cholera for a meeting of the Epidemiological Society on 4 December 1854. Part of this presentation included a map for which he has become famous and which is used as an example of his ground-breaking work. Snow has often been mistakenly credited with the invention of the disease map, but in fact they had been used for some time, even to chart the progress of the plague.[52] The map that Snow used at the Epidemiological Society meeting had in fact been drawn by Edmund Cooper, an engineer working for the Metropolitan Commission of Sewers. Cooper's map already contained short black lines to indicate where the 574 deaths had occurred, which Snow improved on by adding more lines to show the proportion of deaths per household. Snow also added circled dots to show the position of the water pumps, in order to illustrate the relationship between these and the highest number of deaths, but he somewhat strangely drew the Broad Street pump in the wrong position. Later this mistake was rectified in the map produced for the 1855 Cholera Inquiry Committee, but his genius stroke was the addition of a line to indicate walking distances to the Broad Street pump. This altered and extended the number of people previously thought to have consumed water from the pump, and who were subsequently infected. The map was to play a crucial part in confirming Snow's waterborne theory and was later used by writers like William T. Sedgwick to illustrate Snow's brilliance.

Snow put together a full report for the St James's Cholera Inquiry Committee and separate reports were also included from Rev Henry Whitehead and the surveyor Jehoshaphat York; the work was completed in July 1855. Snow was conscious that this paper was another opportunity to prove his cholera theory, but he knew that case studies and accurate statistics were also crucial. As Tom Koch rightly observed in a 2013 essay on Snow, 'It is about convincing others of the correctness of an idea through a methodology all will accept using data everyone can trust.'[53]

Snow described in detail 48 individual cases of people who had died from cholera after drinking water straight from the Broad Street pump. Both Snow and Whitehead in his own report, emphasised that the local Soho population only boiled the water stored in their domestic cisterns to make tea. If cold water was required, they obtained it from the pump. Initially Whitehead had been sceptical towards the theory that the pump was the source of the outbreak, but in January 1855 Snow gave him a copy of his newly published *On the Mode of Communication of Cholera*, which made Whitehead more sympathetic to Snow's ideas. Whitehead's own door-to-door enquiries eventually convinced him that Snow was probably right:[54]

> *'I happened to be studying the Registrar's returns ... when my eye suddenly fell upon the following entry:*
> *"At 40, Broad Street, 2nd September, a daughter, aged*

*five months, exhaustion after an attack of Diarrhea* [sic]
*four days previous to death."*

'*I knew the case and had recorded the date of death, but
somehow had neglected to inquire about the date of attack
... I suppose, because it was the case of an infant. Neither
had it occurred to me that the child might have been ill all
the week. I immediately went to the house and ascertained
from the mother...that the child was attacked on Monday
28th August, and that the dejections at first were abundant,
but ceased on Wednesday 30th August ... she told me that
the dejections were collected in napkins, which, on being
removed, were immediately steeped in pails, the water
from which was poured partly into a sink in the back yard,
and partly into a cesspool in the front area.*' [55]

The resulting hypothesis from Whitehead's assertion was that the
water in the well of the Broad Street pump had been tainted by the
cholera infested nappies of the baby who had died. The infant's father
would also die of cholera, but the baby, or rather her mother's actions,
would be deemed to have caused the outbreak.

Medical historians Vinten et al note that in his report, Whitehead
refers to the surname of family in question as beginning with 'L.'[56]
The only candidates enumerated in the 1851 Census who fit this
criteria in Broad Street are Thomas Lewis, a police constable, aged
46, and his wife Sarah, aged 40, both born in Northamptonshire. Like
many others, they had probably migrated to London hoping for a
brighter future. The role of a London police constable had recently
been redefined, following the Metropolitan Police Act of 1829, and
Thomas Lewis would have been one of London's first 'bobbies' or
'peelers'.

There is no record of exactly when Thomas and Sarah may have
arrived in London, however, their ages and other records suggest that
it was probably in the early 1830s. The first address recorded for them
is Thomas Street, in the parish of St George's Hanover Square, and
they moved to at least two more addresses before finally settling at 40
Broad Street. Frequent house moves were not uncommon for the

working classes and are likely to have been the result of fluctuating rents and Thomas's work.

The couple had at least four children: Anne (1835), Thomas (1838), Elizabeth Ann (1840), and last of all Frances (1854), who was born at Broad Street. Elizabeth Ann was not mentioned in any of the Cholera Inquiry Committee reports. However, in a letter, local surgeon, Dr Rogers, who attended the sick Frances, described the fate of a son, who cannot be traced in genealogical records. That child may have been erroneously described and could have been Elizabeth, though it is possible that the Lewis family had more children who had died during infancy, as Rogers notes Sarah's poor health and difficulties during pregnancy, which could explain the gaps between births.

Following the cholera outbreak in 1854 and the deaths of Frances and Thomas, Sarah and her daughter Anne continued to live at 40 Broad Street, though in the 1861 Census Thomas was enumerated at 236 Regent Street, working for Messrs William Jones and Company as a porter. W. Jones and Co. were manufacturers of military buttons and gold lacework, and purportedly suppliers to Queen Victoria and The Prince of Wales.[57] In 1861 Sarah and Anne are noted as working as laundresses.

Yet was Frances Lewis the true source of the cholera outbreak? In 1855 Henry Whitehead submitted further evidence to the St James's Cholera Inquiry Committee from correspondence received from the physician who had attended the family, Dr Rogers:

> 'It was born, I believe, in April 1854; and was attacked with a Diarrhoea in the June following; its evacuations were pale and slimy, sour and offensive; it was under treatment for about five days; it continued pretty well till the 14th of August, when it had a similar attack, which however gave way to treatment in two or three days, but on the morning of Monday the 28th of August I was sent for ... and found it again suffering from another attack of Diarrhoea, but now accompanied with sickness, so that but little medicine or food could be retained its dejections were pale, slimy, and watery, smelt very offensive; the

*mother tells me they were now and then of a mixed greenish and cream colour; this state of purging and sickness continued till Wednesday (30th). I never saw, that I can remember, what might be taken for Cholera stools, – she never looked bluish, had no cramps, there was no cold stage or collapse, nor subsequent fever, and she always passed her urine which stained the napkins.'* [58]

If this evidence is accurate, then Frances Lewis may not have died of Asiatic cholera. Her death certificate also gives the cause of death as 'Exhaustion after an attack of Diarrhoea four days previous to Death.'[59] The child's symptoms were not those of the severest form of the disease, but the Cholera Inquiry Committee responded that young children did not always suffer from the same symptoms as adults and that her diarrhoea was probably 'choleraic,' in other words a form of cholera.[60]

Snow needed proof that the water from the Broad Street pump was the single source of the cholera outbreak, and the death of Frances Lewis and the conclusions of the committee were crucial for him to establish his hypothesis that cholera is a waterborne disease. The survey conducted by Jehoshaphat York had indicated that the well and drains underneath number 40 Broad Street were permeable, potentially allowing infectious matter to enter the water supply; any contamination of the pump from further afield would be impossible for Snow to prove. A letter concerning the well at Broad Street on September 1854 to the *Medical Times and Gazette*, gives an insight to Snow's concerns:

*'The pump-well in Broad Street is from 28 to 30 feet in depth, and the sewer, which passes a few yards from it, is 22 feet below the surface. This sewer proceeds from Marshall-street, where some cases of cholera had occurred before the great outbreak.*

*'I am of opinion that the contamination of the water of the pump-wells of large towns is a matter of vital importance. Most of the pumps in this neighbourhood yield*

*water that is very impure and I believe that it is merely to the accident of the cholera evacuations not having passed along the sewers nearest to the wells that many localities in London near a favourite pump have escaped a catastrophe similar to that which has just occurred in this parish.'[61]*

In his report to the Cholera Inquiry Committee, Whitehead also seems to have originally had doubts that Frances Lewis could be the source of contamination:

*' ... an infant, whose mother emphatically denies that it ever tasted of the pump water, assigning as a reason a decided objection to this water on the part of her husband, who was himself fatally seized with Cholera on the 8th of September, being almost the last person who was attacked, either fatally or not, in this street. He of course was no drinker of the pump water.'[62]*

Whitehead then mentions another case which may have been the source of the outbreak but had been dismissed:

*' ... the third fatal attack ... that of August 30th was the case of a lad who went to Bayswater on Saturday August 26th, returning Monday the 28th. The family with whom he resided in Broad Street are positive in their assertion that he never drank of the pump water. the precise hour of his attack was 5 a.m.. At noon, the same day, he was sent back to Bayswater. It is worthy of notice that his mother and sister (at Bayswater) were also seized the following evening and died before the end of the week.'[63]*

At the time when the Bayswater boy was in Broad Street, contamination may not yet have occurred, so it is irrelevant whether or not he drank the pump water there. However, if he was already infected with cholera, then his faeces may have entered the privy at number 40 Broad Street and contaminated the well. Snow did not discuss this case or any other that may have raised the question of outside contamination, as this would not have helped to progress his argument.

In the Cholera Inquiry Committee's report, data on cholera deaths for the period 29 July 1854 to 14 October 1854 indicates that the progress of the disease throughout London followed a similar pattern to the Broad Street area, suggesting that they were part of the same outbreak:

| Date | London deaths | St James's deaths |
|------|---------------|-------------------|
| 29 July: | London: 133 | St James's: 0 |
| 5 August: | London: 399 | St James's: 1 |
| 12 August: | London: 644 | St James's: 5 |
| 19 August: | London: 729 | St James's: 12 |
| 26 August: | London: 847 | St James's: 6 |
| 2 September: | London: 1287 | St James's: 78 |
| 9 September: | London: 2050 | St James's: 287 |
| 16 September: | London: 1549 | St James's: 67 |
| 23 September: | London: 1284 | St James's: 19 |
| 30 September: | London: 754 | St James's: 7 |
| 7 October: | London: 411 | St James's: 1 |
| 14 October: | London: 249 | St James's: 0 [64] |

Frances Lewis may have contracted a mild form of cholera, but the disease may also have been brought in from outside of the area or by effluent from other interconnected drains. The survey and resulting report undertaken by Jehoshaphat York discusses the state of the drains leading from number 40 Broad Street, but not the main sewer. The drains were in a very poor state and effluent from number 40 could easily have leaked into the well. The drain connecting the shared privy and cesspool to the sewer ran right alongside the well, and York was in no doubt that both were leaking – the condition of the soil around the well led him to the same conclusion.

However, in September 1854 the main sewer in Broad Street had been inspected by the engineer Edmund Cooper for his report to the Metropolitan Commission of Sewers. He had noted that the pipe running along Broad Street between Marshall Street and Cambridge Street (today's Lexington Street) had been newly constructed in 1851, but he does not reveal whether or not it was fit for purpose. The old drain still in use, running to Berwick Street from west to east, terminated very close to the well that supplied the Broad Street pump with water. This pipe was certainly not in a good state of repair, and as Cooper explained:

> 'Broad-street, a straight street, 50 feet wide, in part of which, between Cambridge-street and Marshall-street, a new sewer was built during the year 1851, with a fall southward towards Windmill-street. In the other portion of Broad-street, no works whatever have of late years been carried on, the sewer there having been built in the year 1823, which discharges itself into Berwick-street, and is entirely unconnected, and perfectly independent, of the sewer above alluded to, built in 1851. The drainage of many of the houses affected in this street is of a very defective character, cesspools no doubt existing at the rear of them, although closet-pans have been fixed.'[65]

Additional information on the pump and the state of the sewers was provided by Edwin Lankester in his 1866 paper, 'Cholera: What is it? And how to Prevent it'. Whilst he agrees with the conclusions of the St James's committee on the source of contamination, he makes further interesting observations. First, he notes that the well in Broad Street was some 25 feet deep, which means that the water within it may well have been exposed to contamination from a wider and deeper, area:

> 'The water percolates into this well through a loose gravel extending for several hundreds of yards to its north and west. All this gravel is covered with streets and houses, and in it have been dug innumerable cesspools and through it

*pass numberless drains – brick drains, rat-eaten, filthy, corrupt drains, and also sewers – bad sewers – some of them in the immediate neighbourhood of the pump only half a brick thick.'*[66]

At the time of John Snow's death in June 1858, despite his numerous reports and speeches, he had failed to achieve widespread acceptance for his theory that cholera was a waterborne disease. One of Snow's most notable critics was Dr Edmund Parkes, whose name also features in the frieze on the London School of Hygiene and Tropical Medicine. Parkes was a highly respected member of the medical establishment, with considerable experience of treating cholera in India and in England, and he had also written extensively on the disease. In the *British and Foreign Medico-Chirurgical Review*, of which he was then the Editor, Parkes gave a critique in April 1855 of Snow's final edition of *On the Mode of Communication of Cholera*. From the outset, Parkes made it clear that whilst he was prepared to consider Snow's argument that cholera was a waterborne disease, he was sceptical that the disease could be 'solely and exclusively so propagated.'[67]

There was much in Snow's text with which Parkes disagreed. He believed Snow's assertion that cholera was entirely local to the alimentary canal to be a mere hypothesis, and countered with his belief that the blood and nervous system still played some part in the infection process. Parkes also felt that Snow arrived too rapidly at conclusions and that he rejected other important contributory factors too swiftly by asserting that cholera could only be waterborne. Parkes argued that Snow had dismissed potential causes such as population density, ventilation and the infection of air prior to any contamination of the water.

Above all, Parkes believed that the evidence supporting Snow's argument was too circumstantial: 'To prove so weighty a fact, we require not only positive, but negative evidence.'[68] Snow's error here, according to Parkes, was that 'He has not been able to prove that all were attacked who drank this water, and that none were attacked who did not drink.'[69] Tom Koch explains that Parkes' view has some validity: ' ... a careful reading of Parkes' concerns insists that the myth of Snow is overstated. Yes, cholera is a waterborne disease. But were we to read Snow's work with attention but without foreknowledge we, too, would find its argument incomplete.'[70]

Parkes concluded his critique thus:

> ' ... *from the positive evidence adduced by Dr. Snow, we were unable to do more than conclude that he had rendered the transmission of cholera by water an hypothesis worthy of inquiry; we cannot draw any other conclusion from his researches on water supply, than that the predisposing effects of impurity of water are also rendered highly probable. We may be mistaken in this, and the evidence which seems weak to us may not be so to others. If so, when additional evidence shall be given, we shall receive it with the greatest pleasure.* '[71]

Edwin Chadwick's assertion, that 'all smell is disease'[72] still rang true with the miasmatist medical elite. Despite Snow's valuable work and the evidence he had presented, most commentators and observers were still unable to abandon their view that the cause of cholera was foul air and not contaminated water. Nonetheless, whatever the cause of the disease, the solution was the same: improved sanitation.

The Bristol physician Dr William Budd was also aware at this time that better sanitation was the way forward. Like Snow, he had vision and persistence, perhaps due to his family's radical political leanings and an upbringing which had encouraged his open-minded approach to life and study. According to Budd's biographer, Michael Dunnill:

> '[Budd was a] *compassionate man with a profound social conscience, he sought to alleviate the lot of the working classes by improving their health and physical welfare as a prerequisite to a better life ...* [His letters] *reveal a mind preoccupied with enquiry into all aspects of medicine, with a profound social awareness of the divide between rich and*

*poor, and a keen desire to relieve suffering. His intellectual
vigour and breadth of interest are astonishing.'* [73]

An insight into Budd's strong social conscience and sense of duty
can also be perceived within his 1849 paper, 'Malignant Cholera: its
cause, mode of propagation, and prevention':

> *'At a time when cholera is destroying hundreds of our
> fellow-creatures daily, and filling the land with mourning,
> it is the duty of every one ... to give them, without delay, all
> the publicity possible ... Entertaining, therefore, a strong
> persuasion that the conclusion is just, I could not acquit my
> conscience without, at once, making public the grounds on
> which it is founded ... how important it is ... for the Rich to
> attend to the physical wants of the Poor. To do this is one
> of our first and plainest duties ... By reason of our common
> humanity, we are all more nearly related here than we are
> apt to think. The members of the great human family are,
> in fact, bound together by a thousand secret ties.'* [74]

Budd, the son of a retired naval surgeon, was born in North Tawton,
Devon, and had enrolled at Edinburgh University in 1837, amongst
those who were to become London's future medical elite. Budd
continued his studies in Paris under Francois-Joseph-Victor Broussais
who, according to Michael Dunnill, had a significant influence on his
research, both in terms of his investigative methods and Broussais'
belief that 'most diseases [were due] to inflammation of the gastrointestinal tract.'[75]

Budd attended further courses in Paris over the years that followed,
including surgical pathology and midwifery.[76] He studied under a
number of influential men, such as the eclectic pathologist Professor
Gabriel Andral and the physician Pierre Louis.[76] Louis was an advocate
of reform and a member of the Idéologues, a group of enlightened
medical men who believed in teaching and research, and whose
approach would also have an impact on Snow.[77] In addition, Louis
may have influenced Budd's belief in preventative medicine.

This background ensured that Budd was open to discussion and to new ideas in medical research. Unlike Snow, he did not dismiss the miasmatists, but rather kept them on side and continued to consider their theory until it could no longer be plausible. Budd was a contagionist and, when his observations on typhoid fever and cholera showed similar causes and effects, he began to realise that disease may be caused by some sort of microorganism, or 'microscopic fungi.'[78] Budd was one of the first to investigate the idea that cholera could be caused by a living organism.[79]

Budd's initial views on cholera were published in 1849, in his *Malignant Cholera: its cause, mode of propagation, and prevention*. It began with the bold pronouncement that Dr Frederick Brittan had discovered that 'peculiar microscopic objects exist constantly in the characteristic "rice-water" discharges of persons affected with Malignant Cholera, and in the atmosphere of infected places.'[80]

Budd, Brittan, Dr Joseph Griffith Swayne and Dr Augustin Pritchard were members of a committee of six[81] appointed by the Bristol Medico-Chirurgical Society in 1849 'for the microscopic observation of subjects connected with cholera.'[82] Budd was keen to point out within his paper that infectious particles were to be found both in the air and in the water, and they had been identified in 'almost every specimen of drinking-water which I was enabled to obtain from Cholera-districts [in Bristol].'[83]

Budd made some important observations in his 1849 paper. He recognised that cholera was 'a living organism of distinct species'[84] and that it had to be ingested into the intestinal canal to take effect. He noted that the disease had unique characteristics, which are 'developed only in the human intestine.'[85] However, Budd differed from Snow in that he did not accept that cholera was solely transmitted through the water but also considered that it might travel in the air and on food. While he understood the role humans played in transmitting cholera from place to place, Budd continued to believe cholera was transmitted through the air, as he could not understand 'its occasional transport over considerable tracts without the intervention of man; its introduction into new countries in spite of quarantine and every other human precaution ... [and] ... the single and casual case.'[86]

However, his initial conclusions were extremely similar to Snow's: Budd agreed that cholera was transmitted through the sewers in water tainted by infected victims, and able to travel even across large distances. Similarly, he believed that the disease was more prevalent at low levels and could also follow the course of streams. Cholera could also infest the waters close to sewage outlets, he asserted, and infect those living on boats who took their water from the river. Budd upheld the contagionist view that people could only become infected if they ate or drank from an infected source, not merely by entering an area where infection was prevalent.[87]

Budd did not take sole credit for his conclusions and he alluded to Snow's 1849 version of *On the Mode of Communication of Cholera*:

> *'Dr. Snow, whose ingenious pamphlet on Cholera fell into my hands while these materials were preparing for publication, has been led, by the consideration of particular instances of some of the facts above alluded to, to the same conclusion as to the part which water plays in the diffusion of the disease. Of being the first to develop and to publish this very important conclusion he must, therefore, have the whole merit.'*[88]

Budd and the Bristol committee were correct in the belief that cholera was caused by a micro-organism. Yet, the structures they identified in greater numbers in the stools of infected patients were a variety of particles and not *Vibrio cholerae*. In early nineteenth century Britain, microscopical investigation was still in its infancy and it was an expensive pursuit. A microscope could cost at least £50 – a large sum of money in those days – and the techniques for fixing and colouring specimens were still limited. Moreover, there was a schism between microscopical investigation and the medical world, as the study was considered more of a hobby for surgeons and clergymen intent on finding a new species rather than the cause of infectious diseases.[89]

In London, Dr Arthur Hill Hassall worked with Snow to try and ascertain if some sort of particle could be responsible for cholera.

Snow gave Hassall some water from the Broad Street pump during his investigations, but the results were not as conclusive as they would have liked:

> *'The water at the time of the cholera contained impurities of an organic nature, in the form of minute whitish flocculi visible on close inspection to the naked eve, as I before stated. Dr. Hassall, who was good enough to examine some of this water with the microscope, informed me that these particles had no organised structure, and that he thought they probably resulted from decomposition of other matter. He found a great number of very minute oval animalcules in the water, which are of no importance, except as an additional proof that the water contained organic matter on which they lived.'* [90]

In Bristol, the Microscopical Society, founded in 1843, counted Budd, Swayne and Pritchard amongst its founder members. The Bristol group stood out from their London colleagues, not least because they were great communicators, were enthusiastic about science and were also all members of the Bristol Medico-Chirurgical Society. There were plenty of opportunities for them to exchange information, and they also had contacts in London. [91]

In these early years of research, it was sufficient that Budd was aware of the nature of cholera for him to develop effective preventative measures. Budd could see that well water, poor sanitation and the densely populated, badly ventilated living conditions within Bristol's tenement dwellings all contributed to ill health. He gave evidence to that effect for the 1845 Second Report of the Commissioners for Inquiring into the State of Large Towns and Populous Districts.

Also key to the development and acceptance of Snow's waterborne theory was Dr John Simon. Prior to his appointment in 1855 as Chief Medical Officer to the new General Board of Health, and whilst he was still Medical Officer of Health for the City of London, Simon had served on the Committee for Scientific Enquiries. This and two other committees had been set up by Sir Benjamin Hall in August 1854 as part of a temporary Board of Health. The Scientific Enquiries committee also included Dr Neil Arnott, Dr William Baly, Dr William Farr, and Professor Richard Owen.

The committee presented its findings in the *Report of the Committee for Scientific Inquiries in Relation to the Cholera-Epidemic of 1854*. Despite Farr's support for Snow's work in Soho, at this time he was still of the opinion that cholera was breathed in through the lungs (in the form of zymotic cholerine particles);[92] Farr did not prevent the report from dismissing the theory that cholera is a waterborne disease:

> '*In explanation of the remarkable intensity of this outbreak within very definite limits, it has been suggested by Dr. Snow, that the real cause of whatever was peculiar in the case lay in the general use of one particular well, situate at Broad Street in the middle of the district, and having (it was imagined) its waters contaminated with the rice-water evacuations of cholera patients.*
>
> '*After careful inquiry, we see no reason to adopt this belief ... The water was undeniably impure with organic contamination; and we have already argued that, if, at the times of epidemic invasion there be operating in the air some influence which converts putrifiable impurities into a specific poison, the water of the locality, in proportion as it contains such impurities, would probably be liable to similar poisonous conversion.*'[93]

Like Farr and Snow, Simon was interested in the statistics showing the variance in mortality rates on the southern banks of the Thames in London for those supplied by water by the Southwark and Vauxhall Water Company and the Lambeth Waterworks. In May 1856 Simon produced a report for the General Board of Health entitled, *Report on the Last Two Cholera-Epidemics of London, as Affected by the Consumption of Impure Water*. Improved statistical information had demonstrated a more distinct difference between mortality rates for those who had ingested water from the different water companies, and

Simon agreed that there was now a far more compelling argument for cholera being a waterborne disease:

> 'In the 24,854 houses supplied by the Lambeth Company, comprising population of about 166,906 persons, there occurred 611 cholera deaths, being at the rate of 37 to every 10,000 living. In the 39,726 houses supplied by the Southwark and Vauxhall Company, comprising a population of about 268,171 persons, there occurred 3,476 deaths, being at the rate of 130 to every 10,000 living.
>
> 'The population drinking dirty water accordingly appears to have suffered 3½ times as much mortality as the population drinking other water'[94]

Simon deduced that in the following epidemic of 1853-4, tainted water had had an even greater effect on mortality rates, and on 26 July 1855 the Southwark and Vauxhall company had moved its intake from Battersea up river to take its supply from the cleaner waters around Hampton.[95] In his report Simon added:

> 'It is, indeed, indispensable for the healthiness of towns, that house-drainage should be universally adopted ... It entirely consists with the facts here set forth to maintain that, under the specific influence which determines an epidemic period, fecalised drinking-water and fecalised air equally may breed and convey the poison; and that this, whether in one vehicle or the other, may be expected to prevail most forcibly against the feeble and ill-nourished parts of a population.'[96]

On 25 June 1856, *The Times* published an article commentating on Simon's report, followed by a response from Snow the next day in which he lamented Simon's inaccuracies and the lack of credit for his own work, which had formed the foundation for Simon's ideas:

*'The population supplied with the impure water of the Southwark and Vauxhall company suffered a mortality from cholera in the late epidemic not merely three and a half times as great as that supplied by the Lambeth Company, but six times as great; and even this fact expresses the influence of the impure water in an inadequate manner, unless the different periods of the epidemic are considered separately.*

*'The inquiry which supplies the matter for Mr. Simon's report was not an original one undertaken during the epidemic, but an additional investigation made under very disadvantageous circumstances after the epidemic was over. Early in the epidemic of 1854 I commenced a personal inquiry respecting every death from cholera which occurred in the districts in which the water supply of the above companies is intermixed.'* [97]

However, it would take more than statistics and scientific observation to prove that cholera was indeed waterborne. Snow died prematurely in June 1858, possibly of a stroke, though his underlying health had previously been poor. His theory was still not widely accepted and he did not live to read of Robert Koch's 1884 discovery of the cholera pathogen, *Vibrio cholerae*. Nonetheless, at the time of his death Snow would have been aware that the weather was particularly warm for the time of year. He may even have noticed the putrid smells emanating from the River Thames – the so-called 'Great Stink', which was to become the next catalyst for sanitary reform.

# CHAPTER 8

# The Stink of Cholera:
# The improvement of London's sewage
# system and Sir Joseph Bazalgette

At the beginning of June 1858, Member of Parliament Darby Griffith asked a question in the House of Commons about the state of the River Thames and whether the gasses emanating from the surface of the water could be dangerous to health.[1] It was suggested that he should speak directly to the Metropolitan Board of Works and questions continued on other matters. Three days later, a letter by Griffith appeared in *The Times* expressing frustration that his idea of constructing a system of drainage and sewage pipes within the banks of the River Thames had been brushed to one side.

Despite John Snow's work in Soho and the acceptance that London's water supply needed to be drawn from purer sources, the professional and medical elite still saw little immediate need to overhaul London's primitive network of sewage and water pipes. There were many reasons why change continued to be obstructed. London was still divided into different districts at this stage, and there was no single body overseeing the capital's future development, (as discussed in Chapter 3). The places that most urgently needed a sanitary infrastructure were the difficult to drain, low-lying areas and these were also some of the most densely populated in the capital. In areas such as Southwark and Lambeth, on the south bank of the Thames, workers' tenements had been hastily erected and built right up to noxious factories and manufacturing premises. Not only were the poor of London deemed less important, but excavation in such areas for the building of a new sewage system would cause significant disruption, particularly from a commercial point of view.

For this reason factory owners were vehemently opposed to change, yet they were caught in the crossfire of the two debates then raging over public health. On the one hand, industrial areas were those most in need of sanitation, but on the other, factories spewed out the noxious smells that many believed caused disease. An additional argument for not overhauling London's sanitary infrastructure was the cost, and there was considerable opposition from the local authorities, property owners and employers to spending such vast sums of money, least of all on the poor.

Within the scientific community there was some support for Snow's theory that cholera was a waterborne disease, but the miasmatist, anti-contagionist view still persisted. One of those who upheld this belief was Dr William Baly, who was appointed physician for Millbank Penitentiary, London's riverside prison, in 1841. Here Baly witnessed at first-hand the suffering of inmates from dysentery and cholera and experimented with various remedies and potential cures. He wrote prolifically and was considered an authority on health and hygiene in prisons.

In much of his research, Baly collaborated with William Withey Gull, a distinguished surgeon who, like Baly, was a Fellow of the Royal College of Physicians. In 1849 Baly and Gull collaborated on the *Report on the Nature and Import of Certain Microscopic Bodies Found in the Intestinal Discharges of Cholera* for the Cholera Committee of the Royal College of Physicians in London. The work began with a discussion of the research into the disease going on in Bristol. Unlike Swayne and Brittan, Baly and Gull had found no tiny particles in their investigations of condensed air. They had, however, observed structures in water from samples provided by Snow and from the cisterns of Millbank Penitentiary, but their conclusions were so varied that they refused to believe in the existence of a specific cholera fungus. Instead, they concluded that 'the bodies found by Messrs. Brittan and Swayne are not the cause of Cholera and have no exclusive connexion with that disease ... the whole theory of the disease which has recently been propounded, is erroneous as far as it is based on the existence of the bodies in question.'[2]

As long as the belief persisted that foul air spread disease, the need for a new sanitation system was not considered a priority by the Government. However, in June 1858 temperatures in London began to soar past 80 degrees. The waters of the Thames were recorded at 62.1 degrees, and unsurprisingly the river began to give off the most obnoxious smell. As 'An Oarsman' complained to *The Times*:

> *'The stinks of our once noble and respected Father Thames are now too nauseous for endurance. I rowed on Saturday from Westminster to the Crabtree in Putney Reach, and there was no intermittence – no cessation – one fatal, horrid, open, deadly cesspool. What is to be done?'*[3]

On 11 June 1858, another question was asked in the House of Commons by a Mr Brady, regarding whether any action had been taken to 'mitigate the effluvium from the Thames ... Hon. members sitting in the committee-rooms and library were scarcely able to bear it.'[4]

Temperatures climbed and, as the Houses of Parliament are situated right on the river, members began to find the stench intolerable:

> *'Some time early in June we assembled in one of the rooms then unoccupied. The day was very warm, and we instinctively glanced at the windows with a look that plainly asked why the free breath of heaven was not suffered to enter. At length a member went over to the window near to him, and flung up a portion of it; but no sooner had he done so than he retreated as if he had received a blow in the face., and in the same moment we all expressed our disgust and loathing by ejaculations of a lively and energetic character ... we felt ourselves half choked and half poisoned ... I do not in the slightest degree exaggerate when I say we might have just as well stood over a filthy cesspool or a putrid drain as have inhaled the air which the noxious gases of the Thames had utterly polluted.'*[5]

Between 1853 and 1854, a Royal Commission on the Corporation of the City of London had proposed to replace the Metropolitan Commission of Sewers with the Metropolitan Board of Works to oversee all public projects in the capital, such as the building of a new sewage system. The Board was not created until March 1855, when the Metropolis Local Management Bill was introduced to Parliament by the Chief Commissioner of Works, Sir Benjamin Hall. The Bill proposed dividing London into the same 36 registration districts used for the 1851 Census.

London would continue to be governed by the local vestries elected by ratepayers. Vestry members would then, in turn, be elected by their peers to represent each area on a new central Metropolitan Board of Works. The vestries and local boards would then be responsible for their local sewer infrastructure, but any work would be overseen by the Metropolitan Board of Works, which was now solely responsible for the building of intercepting sewers linking each area of the capital.[6]

The Metropolitan Board of Works commenced its task to improve London's drains and sewers on 1 January 1856, under the chairmanship of John Thwaites. By the end of the month, Joseph Bazalgette had been appointed as Chief Engineer to the Board, following his position as Chief Engineer to the Metropolitan Sewers Commission. As previously discussed in Chapter 3, the creation of the Board and the appointment of Bazalgette was the culmination of many years of confusion and argument. By the summer of 1858, Bazalgette's plans were in place but there were still hurdles to cross. One of the difficulties of the Metropolis Local Management Act was that both plans for a new sewer network and any expenditure over £50,000 required the approval of the Commissioners of Public Works and Public Buildings; expenditure over £100,000 would need approval by Parliament.[7]

Rather than ensuring that work was carefully considered and properly thought through, these restrictions simply slowed down the process. Sir Benjamin Hall took on the engineering consultants Captain Douglas Galton, James Simpson and Thomas E. Blackwell, all of whom had considerable experience, but even they could not agree on a final plan. The nub of the problem was probably the enormous cost and whether additional expenses should be covered by central government or local ratepayers. A change of government at the beginning of 1858 and the replacement of Sir Benjamin Hall by Lord John Manners did not help matters. The catalyst for change was the stink of the river, which provided MPs with a visceral reminder of the problem that summer, as observed in a letter to *The Times*:

> *'Sir, – Ten days' hot weather is likely to do more for the purification of the Thames than ten years of commissions, reports, blue-books, and all the intricate machinery of proving "officially" the existence of an evil of which everyone is "practically" cognizant.'* [8]

On 15 July 1858, the Leader of the House, Benjamin Disraeli, introduced the Metropolis Local Management Amendment Act, extending the powers of the Board of Works and enabling it to speed up the commencement of the new sewer system.[9] In doing so Disraeli swept away the financial and legal barriers preventing the Board from progressing, and once the act became law, on 2 August 1858, the Board was finally able to move ahead.

Bazalgette's design was as ambitious, and potentially as disruptive for Londoners as the building of the London Underground and Crossrail. It was also very expensive, with an estimated initial cost of £2,836,601, though the eventual total would rise to a staggering £4,107,277. This was considerably more than the estimated £1.3 million cost of building the first stretch of the London Underground between Farringdon and Paddington in 1862.[10] Disraeli's amendment had provided the security to borrow up to £3 million to build the new sewage system, which could be repaid over the next 40 years; in July 1863 Parliament and the Exchequer granted permission to borrow the additional funds required.[11]

The basis of Bazalgette's plan was a series of intercepting sewers running parallel to the River Thames, which would discharge waste far away from London into the sea. The sewers would be fed by a network of drains, and smaller pipes and liquid waste would be carried by gravity to two outfall sites: to the north at Barking, and to the south at Crossness near Plumstead. The northern section would require the building of three main intercepting sewers at three different levels. The first and highest would run from Hampstead Heath to Old Ford, Stratford, the second from Kensal Green to Old Ford, with a branch to Piccadilly and another parallel to Gray's Inn Road.

The third and lowest level sewer was perhaps to become the most well-known. This was to begin at Pimlico and would follow the northern bank of the river underneath a newly constructed Victoria Embankment. The sewer would continue towards Tower Hill and Bow, with two branches to the Isle of Dogs and Homerton. The difficulty of London's low-lying geography would be overcome at Abbey Mills in Stratford, where a pumping station would lift waste almost 40 feet, to join sewage from the high and middle sewers. It is testament to Bazalgette's vision and engineering skills that Abbey Mills is still operated by Thames Water.[12] Today a Grade I listed building, and considered by many a Gothic cathedral to sewage, it has become a tourist attraction in recent years.

To the west of London Bazalgette had originally planned a reservoir for waste at Fulham, as the western side of London towards Hammersmith was too low for waste to feed into the rest of the system by gravity. Objections to this idea in 1863 caused Bazalgette to change direction and, whilst it would cost a further £180,000, it was decided to include another pumping station at Chelsea.[13] Bazalgette's design for the southern area of the Thames included a high level sewer from Clapham High Street to Deptford, incorporating as a branch the ancient River Effra, which had become a filthy and notorious open sewer. The low level section would run from Putney High Street to Deptford, with a branch at Bermondsey. Another pumping station was to be built at Deptford, where the two sewers met, lifting waste some 20 feet at this point up to the outfall sewer and on to Crossness.

All projects had to be approved by the Board of Works and all contracts were put out to tender, publicised through advertisements in periodicals like *The Builder*. Most of the work for Bazalgette's plan was undertaken by the established civil engineering companies of William Webster, Thomas Brassey, and George Furness.[14] The latter two had some considerable experience in the building of railways. It is unclear whether the noted builder Samuel Baker and his firm Baker and Sons of Rochester, Kent were also involved in construction. In his account of the project, which is drawn on here, historian Stephen Halliday remarks that Baker was in negotiations with Bazalgette during an unpleasant period. At this time, the employment of George Furness by Bazalgette and rumours of possible financial corruption were under scrutiny by the Board. There had been speculation that Bazalgette's choice of contractors was coloured by the commission he received. However, the Committee of Enquiry set up to look into the matter exonerated Bazalgette, who subsequently reassured the Board that he had not chosen Baker and Sons because they had wanted to impose an unacceptable arbitration clause as a condition of their employment.[15]

Baker's biographer and descendant, Michael Baker, is not aware of any involvement of the Rochester company in the building of the sewers. The firm worked on many projects with the architect Robert Smirke, who married into the family, and by the 1860s the Bakers had already helped to complete some of London's most prestigious buildings, most notably, the dome and Reading Room at the British Library. In 1873, Baker and Sons won the contract to build the Natural History Museum, but problems with the supply of terracotta tiles and an escalation in costs caused the company's eventual collapse. However, between the building of the Reading Room and the Natural History Museum there is a gap of some years during which they may have tendered for, and perhaps built, part of the sewage network. The work would certainly have been of the highest quality.[16]

With a view to saving time and money, Bazalgette issued a series of contracts to each builder, depending on the type of work to be undertaken. A separate set of drawings was used for each contract, superimposed on top of the Ordnance Survey map. These, along with material specifications, were also inspected by a quantity surveyor. Whilst London's Crossrail tunnels have been constructed using giant boring machines, much of Bazalgette's sewer system, like parts of London's underground railway, was built using the cut and cover method. Many of the sewers were situated under main roads and this method caused significant disruption, but tunnelling was more expensive and only used for sewers situated more than 30 feet underground.

Eighty-two miles of sewers were to be built in all, providing London with a new modern underground infrastructure. In addition, 165 miles of the old sewer network was reconstructed and 1,100 miles of local sewers were built by district vestries. Every foot of the work was overseen and checked meticulously by Joseph Bazalgette. Crossness was opened by the Prince of Wales, the future King Edward VII, in April 1865. However, work was not completed there until 1867 and – despite the 1866 outbreak of cholera in the East End – construction at Abbey Mills and in the western section of the system was finished in 1868.[17]

Perhaps inspired by Member of Parliament Darby Griffith, Bazalgette's plan included three new major embankments on the River Thames: to the north the Victoria and to the south the Chelsea and the Albert. In fact the idea had already been put forward by Sir Christopher Wren, and the nineteenth century painter John Martin had also considered such a scheme.[18] The Victoria Embankment, which would incorporate the land occupied by the Houses of Parliament, would be the grander of the three and would conceal service pipes and a tunnel for the underground railway, as well as the intercepting sewer.

Yet, whilst so much thought was given to the north side of the river, the banks directly opposite at Lambeth and Southwark, which were arguably more in need of a modern sewage system, were considered less important. Lambeth and Southwark were the areas of London worst affected by cholera during the 1848-9 outbreak. In Lambeth alone around 2,000 people died out of a population of just under 116,000. Most of the deaths occurred in the waterfront area, where Dr John Snow had observed residents taking their drinking water directly from the river.

The land was low-lying, crammed with noxious industries and thousands of jerry-built tenements, which were arranged around courtyards and interspersed with narrow alleyways:

*'A street called Upper and Lower Fore-street ... cut off by the gas works belonging to the Vauxhall Company. In this*

*street are bone-boilers, soap-makers, tallow-melters ... and other equally unwholesome trades. A large number of poor families live in this street, in little low houses, the rooms of which are scarcely high enough for a person to stand upright in; scarcely any of these houses have privies, the dust heap appearing to be the common receptacle for all filth. The tide from the Thames flows up to the doors, and when it recedes it leaves all the filth from its banks opposite the houses, the stench from which when it dries is fearful. Behind it ... Princes-street ... literally studded with courts and alleys, all densely inhabited by poor persons ... bone-houses ... soap boilers ... grease-works ... When the bone-boilers are at work, which is almost every day, it is next to impossible for a stranger to pass through the street without being compelled to vomit ... About 800 poor families live on this immediate spot.'[19]*

Industry had flourished in Lambeth since the early years of the nineteenth century. However, the waterfront had become particularly squalid in the 1840s, when the railway line from Nine Elms to Waterloo Station had effectively cut the area off. Bazalgette's plan involved a radical solution. Rather than re-develop the waterfront to provide proper housing and new factory buildings, the decision was taken to replace the entire stretch with the Albert Embankment. The structure was, and still is, an important flood barrier and an essential traffic artery between Lambeth and Vauxhall Bridges, though the original structure stopped some 1,000 feet short of Vauxhall Bridge due to lack of funds.[20] Perhaps most important of all, the view from the Houses of Parliament, which was situated directly opposite, was considerably enhanced.

Of all London's boroughs, Lambeth was, perhaps, most urgently in need of decent sanitation, yet, the Albert Embankment was not incorporated into Bazalgette's sewer plan and his drawings show that, unlike the Victoria Embankment, it did not contain the same infrastructure of sewers, pipes and tunnels.

The 1861 the Lambeth Bridge Act paved the way for the

construction of the Albert Embankment. The ancient horse ferry was replaced by a new bridge in 1862 connecting Church Street on the southern bank to Market Street, (today's Horseferry Road), in Westminster. A new Waterloo Station was built on the site of the old St Thomas' Hospital, which moved further up the road to Lambeth. The money that the hospital paid for this land helped to offset the cost of the Embankment, and building work started in 1864, following approval from Parliament.[21]

The Albert Embankment was seen as a solution to Lambeth's problems and was the first of the riverside embankments to open in 1868, with the official opening on 24 November 1869. The ceremony was conducted by John Thwaites, Chairman of the Metropolitan Board of Works, accompanied by Bazalgette and the architect to the Board, George Vulliamy. The ceremony was not particularly grand and included a band, which played 'See the Conquering Hero Comes', a piece composed by Handel to celebrate the Duke of Cumberland's defeat of the Jacobite Rebellion.

In contrast, when the Victoria Embankment was opened by the Prince of Wales in July 1870, various members of the royal family were in attendance, as well as most of the House of Commons and foreign ambassadors. The event was watched by some 10,000 ticket holders from stands and music was played by the Grenadier and Coldstream Guards.[22] The Chelsea Embankment, which incorporated the main low level West London sewer, was subsequently completed in 1874. It was opened on 9 May of the same year by the Chairman of the Metropolitan Board of Works, Lieutenant Colonel Sir James MacNaughton Hogg, and the Duke and Duchess of Edinburgh. The Duke was Queen Victoria's second son, Prince Alfred, who had married the Grand Duchess Maria Alexandrovna, the daughter of the Emperor of Russia, in 1874. A booklet published to commemorate the opening stated that the Chelsea Embankment had cost an estimated £134,000 'exclusive of the expenditure for purchase of property and compensations.'[23]

Bazalgette also designed bridges at Putney and Battersea, and a steam ferry which traversed the Thames between North and South Woolwich. He was responsible for raising the levels of the banks of all the wharves and banks along 40 miles of the Thames to prevent flooding. At home and abroad he was involved with very many other projects, including the planning of the Blackwall Tunnel at Greenwich.[24] Bazalgette was knighted by Queen Victoria in 1874 and received tremendous acclaim for his work, which had transformed London, although his work on the sewage network was not completed until the following year.[25]

The building of London's new system had taken a tremendous toll on Bazalgette's health, just as it had on that of his predecessor, Forster. Bazalgette was responsible for every aspect of the network's construction, including disputes and unproven allegations of financial corruption. Towards the end of 1869, the Board of Works ordered him to take three months' leave, appointing John Grant in his place, but Bazalgette could only stay away for a few weeks. In his final years he was plagued with asthma, and he died at his home in Wimbledon in 1891, aged 72.[26]

The building of London's new sewage system had taken almost 20 years to complete and cost more than any other engineering project of its time. Work has continued to maintain and extend Bazalgette's system, and today major engineering projects, such as new sewage works and tunnels to deal with overflow, are being developed to cope with London's expanding population.[27] Despite the limitations which have occurred more recently as a result of population growth and changes in weather patterns affecting rainfall, Bazalgette's system transformed the health of London and has been of the greatest benefit to public health, providing clean water and helping to eradicate waterborne diseases like cholera.

CHAPTER 9

# Cholera Returns:
# The 1866 East End cholera outbreak
# and the *Princess Alice* disaster

A fourth cholera pandemic began to spread from the Bay of Bengal in 1863. Its progress was similar to that of the previous outbreaks, along trade routes and proliferating at every harbour or port. The introduction of steamships meant that journey times had become faster, facilitating the spread of disease from one densely populated coast to another.

During this period, as Britain's Empire was expanding, it was essential to find a faster way to reach India and the Far East than the route around the Cape of Good Hope. This was not just for the transportation of goods, but also to speed up communication by providing a more effective postal system. The Red Sea was seen as the solution and the East India Company commissioned Robert Moresby and Thomas Elwon to chart this hazardous stretch of water.[1]

In the 1840s, the overland route across Egypt, linking the Red Sea to the Mediterranean was established by the naval lieutenant, Thomas Fletcher Waghorn, of Chatham, Kent, as explained by Medway historian Dr Andrew Ashbee:

> '[Waghorn] ... *put the final part of the jigsaw into place, in particular the 84 mile trek across the desert from Cairo to Suez. Waghorn's principal aim was to speed the mails between England and India; passengers were secondary to this. Nevertheless their numbers continued to increase, in spite of many discomforts.* '[2]

Since 1837 the job of carrying the Royal Mail between Britain and Gibraltar had been undertaken by the steam ships of the Peninsular Steam Navigation Company, or P&O, which was based at Southampton. Once the route from Alexandria to the Red Sea had been established by Waghorn, additional legs were set up by P&O between Gibraltar and Malta, Malta and Corfu, and Corfu and Alexandria. Post and passengers would then travel overland to Suez and then in East India Company ships to Calcutta on the Bay of Bengal.[3] By the 1860s the route had become the maritime highway between India and Britain. In 1864 when cholera arrived in Aden, at the southern tip of the Red Sea, it was able to spread north swiftly, both by land and sea, reaching Mecca, just under 500 miles inland from the Red Sea coast, in April the following year. Here it infected Muslim pilgrims, killing some 15,000 over the course of the outbreak; similar devastation was repeated in Egypt and Naples.[4] Cholera spread through Europe once again and from Britain it was transported to the West Indies and by emigrant ships from Liverpool to the United States.

Waghorn had not just created a faster and more direct route for the postal service from the Bay of Bengal to Southampton, he had also unwittingly created a highway for cholera. Southampton was one of the disease's first ports of call during the Indian Summer of September 1865 and its arrival was announced in newspapers such as *The Times*:

*'We are informed on most unquestionable authority that a decided and undoubted case of Asiatic cholera, with a fatal result, has occurred in Southampton. The victim was a man named Rose, about 30 years of age, residing in Brewhouse-court, Brewhouse-lane, who died on Sunday, about 36 hours from his first attack, the symptoms at every stage being those of the most virulent form of this dreadful disease ... the town of Southampton is in direct communication, by means of the mail steamers, with the Mediterranean, and only four days from Gibraltar, where the cholera now prevails, and at which port these steamers call, every possible sanitary precaution should at once be taken to guard the health, not only of the inhabitants of Southampton, but of the country at large.'*[5]

At the time, according to the General Register Office, the population of Southampton was just over 53,000, and between the initial outbreak and Saturday, 27 October there were 34 fatalities from cholera;[6] by November 1866, 98 deaths had been registered.[7]

Following the initial outbreak, factors such as sensible local sanitation measures and a greater awareness of the disease by the authorities and the general population appeared to have controlled a more widespread outbreak, though cooling seasonal temperatures may also have played a part. Reports in the newspapers were optimistic that Britain had been spared another epidemic. However, by May of the following year reports of cholera cases were on the increase again, and the Quarantine Department of the Privy Council considered taking measures to protect Britain's ports. Southampton's Sanitary Board sent a deputation to London to meet with Dr John Simon, Chief Medical Officer to the Privy Council. The Southampton deputation explained that the September outbreak had shown that once cholera had arrived in a port it was impossible to contain the disease, but should further cases arrive in Southampton by ship, then the city was well prepared to fight any infection:

> *'All the courts and alleys are limewashed, lodginghouses cleansed or closed, gullies and drains trapped and deodorized, all the nuisances reported by the house-to-house visitation at the close of last year have been removed ... and a permanent staff of one medical officer charged with the health of the town, one principal inspector of nuisances, and four assistant inspectors, who devote their time to sanitary measures, are actively engaged in the important duties, in addition to the services of Mr. Wiblin, the Government superintendent of quarantine.'*[8]

The legislation of the preceding years seemed to be taking effect, moreover, local sanitary committees, such as Southampton's, had grasped the link between filth and disease, and perhaps even the possibility that cholera was a waterborne disease.

However, on 10 June 1866, the following announcement appeared in *The Times* regarding a steamer which had arrived in Southampton laden with mail from Bombay and several passengers:

> '*The Peninsular and Oriental Steam Navigation Company's steamer* Poonah *has arrived here with 108 passengers ... In consequence of a case of cholera having occurred on board ... yesterday morning which terminated fatally in nine hours, Dr. Wiblin ... communicated with the local authorities in accordance with the Order of Council ... the surgeon of the ship, Dr. Chapman,* [said] *that the case was one of English cholera, and that the passengers and crew were all in good health.*'[9]

It rapidly emerged that certain members of the crew were suffering from full-blown Asiatic cholera, but by this time they had disembarked and were dispersed throughout the city. Chief Medical Officer John Simon asked Dr Edmund Parkes to visit Southampton. Parkes had worked in India as a military surgeon, before setting up a practice in London in 1845. In 1855 he had been sent by the government to the Crimea during the war, to establish a relief hospital at Renkioi in the Dardanelles.[10] Parkes had seen cholera in all its forms, he was experienced, and had written several papers on the matter; he was also well aware of the work of Dr John Snow.

Parkes reported on the outbreak in Southampton for the Privy Council[11] and the work was reproduced in *The British and Foreign Medico-Chirurgical Review*:

> '*On the 10th June* [1866] *the Peninsular and Oriental Steamship* Poonah *arrived from Alexandria, Malta, and Gibraltar. On the voyage home the crew and passengers enjoyed perfect health until two days before arriving at Southampton, when several men became ill with severe diarrhoea, and one died of cholera.*'

Parkes noted that the outbreak had been caused by dirty water which the ship had taken on in Gibraltar, where cholera was already raging. The outbreak had begun with a fireman on board who had drunk from the tainted water supply on 8 June and Parkes went on to describe the man's symptoms, which began the following morning: ' ... he was seized with vomiting, purging, and cramps; he became cold and pulseless, and died in nine hours.'

The man died the following day, 9 June, and then over the next few days up to 13 more firemen fell ill. Parkes reported what happened when they arrived in port at Southampton:

> 'None of these men reported themselves to the medical officer, as they were afraid of being detained on board, and they all landed at Southampton and dispersed themselves over the town on the 10th and 11th of June. They were seen by several medical men, who diagnosed the disease as the severest choleraic diarrhoea ... Edward Palmer, one of the firemen in the same watch as the man who had died on board, went to his home, in a very clean and airy situation, on Sunday, June 10th.'

Later that day or the next Palmer began to suffer from diarrhoea, which became progressively worse over the next few days. Parkes described how the man usually went to the outside privy but sometimes used a pot in the room where he slept with his wife and son. The situation then became worse, as Parkes went on to describe:

> 'On Wednesday, June 13th, his child, a boy, aged about three years, and previously in perfect health, was suddenly taken ill at 10 a.m. with violent vomiting, purging, and cramps; he soon became very cold, and died at 4 p.m. The child was seen by several medical men, who were satisfied that the case was one of cholera. On the Thursday Palmer himself became worse; the eyes were sunken, the hands shrivelled; he passed no urine; and he died on Friday, June 15th.'

The two cases were isolated and for this reason Parkes concluded that the cholera must have been communicated to the child when the father's illness was at the diarrhoeal stage and before any cholera symptoms had begun. Parkes concluded:

> 'It can scarcely be doubted that all the men who landed from the Poonah with so-called diarrhoea suffered from the same disease ... and that this disease was cholera. This being admitted, there can be no doubt that the dejecta of cholera in large quantities must have passed from eight or ten persons into the sewers of the town, and in this way there is reason to believe that cholera was introduced into Southampton.'

Following the death of Edward Palmer and his son, there were four more cases of cholera in Southampton between 12 June and 6 July. Then, on 5 July the number of deaths rapidly increased, to around 35 to 37 before 17 July, with the highest mortality in the low-lying and most deprived areas of the city. Parkes added that during August, September and October the epidemic persisted with a few cases, but the worst was over. He then went on to explain how he believed the outbreak had spread:

> 'The poison was probably disseminated through the sewers. At the lower part of the town the sewers are ill ventilated; the sewage accumulates, and gases are often forced into the houses. Just before the outbreak the pumping of sewage had been discontinued while the sewers were being cleansed. The pumping was resumed at the commencement of July, several tons of offensive sewage being daily poured down an open conduit into the outlet sewer.'[12]

In 1855 Parkes had criticised Dr John Snow and, whilst he does not rule out the possibility that others factors were at work, there was now no question in his mind that cholera was a waterborne disease which was being spread through the sewers.

Following the outbreak in Southampton, in April 1866 cholera made its appearance in Bristol. Here too it was contained, to a large extent thanks to the preventative work undertaken by Dr William Budd and his colleague Dr David Davies, the local Medical Officer of Health. Budd had played an important role in improving Bristol's water supply. His work on typhoid as well as cholera had convinced him, like Snow, that clean water was essential for the health of Bristol's population. He gave persuasive evidence to this effect to the Health of Towns Commission (1843-8),[13] contributing to their 1845 inquiry into the state of urban areas.

In 1845 Budd became one of the first directors of the newly established Bristol Waterworks Company and in this capacity he was able to play a part in organising a new infrastructure for the city, stipulating the necessity for a clean water supply brought into the city under pressure that would be free of sewage contamination. The new scheme was to be a complicated endeavour, involving the paying off of competitors and requiring the passage of a bill through parliament; Royal Assent was given in July 1847. To design and oversee the project Budd brought in the experienced engineer James Simpson, who had worked on many other schemes around the country, eventually including the new Lambeth Waterworks site at Thames Ditton. In Bristol reservoirs were subsequently constructed on the Downs, Brandon Hill and outside the city, and 45 miles of pipe were put in place.[14]

In 1866 the first recorded case of cholera in Bristol was thought to be that of a mariner named Henry Thomas, who was travelling from Rotterdam via London. Thomas started suffering from the disease on the train journey from London and died within 18 hours of arriving in Bristol.[15] Budd and Davies attended the sick man and on his death they acted swiftly, informing William Farr at the General Register Office in London of their actions.

Bristol was an important port and, with its many insanitary and densely populated tenement dwellings, the city was vulnerable to cholera. Budd and Davies immediately began a series of preventative measures. With the help of donations from wealthy friends, they got together a group of 28 women who were each given a district to supervise, overseeing the thorough cleaning of houses, privies, drains and sewers of anyone suspected of having cholera. The women ensured that the bedding used by infected cholera victims was destroyed, and that the handles of water pumps in areas affected by the disease were removed. In addition, the Bristol Board of Guardians issued instructions to residents to clean their privies every night and morning for as long as cholera persisted and depots were also set up around the city to distribute free disinfectant. The 1866 outbreak was successfully contained and there were only 29 deaths in the city.[15]

Cholera broke out in many towns and cities across Britain in 1866, including: Edinburgh, Llanelly, Birmingham, Manchester, Salford, Sheffield, Leeds, Hull, Exeter, Weymouth, Portland, Dorchester, Newcastle, Glasgow, Gateshead, North Shields, Sunderland, Durham and Liverpool. In May 1866, *The Times* reported:

> *'The disease in its epidemic character may at any moment be upon us. But the truth is that its course since its appearance in Europe last Midsummer has been marked by none of the usual characteristics ... The cholera of 1865 was not like the Cholera of 1849 or 1832. It was less of an exotic pestilence and more of an ordinary epidemic.'*[16]

If cholera had now become a less dangerous disease, as the report suggests, then it was because some areas of the country, like Bristol, were better prepared than others. There were greater efforts to contain the disease, to clean infected areas, and an increased awareness that cholera may have something to do with tainted water, as this extract from *The Times* illustrates:

> *'Last week it was noticed ... there had been a violent outbreak of cholera in the seaport of North Shields, and that the cause of it was imputed to be the impurity of the water furnished to the districts where the disease prevailed. Within a fortnight there have been fully 100 deaths.'*[17]

However, as the situation in South Shields shows, an increased awareness of how the disease travelled was not always enough to prevent cholera from spreading. Poor living conditions and sanitation in many of the poorest areas had still not been fully addressed. One such deprived place was the East End of London and here cholera broke out with characteristic violence, though initially there was relatively little concern. One of the earliest deaths recorded occurred on 31 May 1866 in Bethnal Green, when the five-year-old son of a warehouseman died just over 24 hours after his symptoms became visible.[18]

Then, in the middle of July, as the weather became much warmer, William Farr noticed a worrying trend, as he informed *The Times*:

> '*Of the 32 deaths from cholera reported in the Registrar-General's returns for the past week it is significant that nearly two-thirds occurred in the eastern districts of the metropolis. Poplar, filled with ill-built and overcrowded houses, returned four deaths; Bethnal-green, the head quarters of London misery and poverty, two deaths from cholera; Limehouse again returned two cases; Ratcliff, Whitechapel, Shoreditch, St. George-in-the-East, one case each.* '[19]

Farr took a keen interest in these emerging statistics and in a supplement which accompanied his 1868 *Annual Report*, he included a full description of the East End outbreak. He noted that cholera cases had started to escalate on Monday, 16 July. Thirty-two deaths had been registered the previous week but by Saturday, 21 July this had risen to 308, and sufferers' symptoms were noted as particularly violent. During this period the weather was extremely hot and reports from local newspapers reveal that in that same week there had been spring tides.[20]

Having been made aware of the effective preventative measures taken by Budd and Davies in Bristol, Farr knew that: 'Immediate measures should be adopted by house-to-house visitation and otherwise to treat the disease in its earliest stage of diarrhoea. And the cholera excretions should be effectually removed or destroyed.'[21] In the following days there were around 868 deaths from cholera in the East End, and the worst affected areas were Bethnal Green, Whitechapel, St George in the East, Stepney, Mile End Old Town and Bow. Farr was still of the opinion that cholera was spread 'through air, contact, and water,'[22] and when he visited the affected area at the beginning of August he noted, 'The air of East London is often charged with impurities, which are undoubtedly noxious.'[23]

The water in the areas worst hit by cholera was supplied by the East London Waterworks Company. The company drew water from the River Lea and the New River, a channel which had been dug in the 1600s to bring fresh spring water from springs in Hertfordshire. The towns of Hertford and Ware discharged sewage into these channels, and whilst that from Ware was not treated at source, the water subsequently passed through 13 filter beds at Lea Bridge over a stretch of 12 acres. Farr regarded the upper reaches of the Lea and the New River as no worse than the Thames, and the areas supplied with water which had been through the filter beds were not affected by cholera. However, from Lea Bridge, water was then fed into a covered reservoir at Old Ford where Farr says, 'The water ... looks perfectly pure. Close by its side, which is well built, flows the tidal end of the Lea, black and full of the foulest impurities.'[24]

It is unclear whether the areas of the East End affected by cholera were supplied with water exclusively from Old Ford, or also from an additional two uncovered reservoirs, one of which 'was recently emptied, and was filled again perhaps by springs or soakage.'[25] What is evident, and as Farr observes, is that the water courses and reservoirs were all connected in some way and there was ample opportunity for cross-contamination:

'At Lea Bridge ... The rest of the water is conveyed down two miles or more of a large iron main to Old Ford, where it is lodged in a small covered underground reservoir, for distribution by three powerful pumping engines: the pipes of Old Ford inosculating freely with those of Lea Bridge, the water system in the pipes sways backwards and *forwards at their juncture according as the waters above or below prevail ... The waters of the aqueduct at Lea Bridge can be passed directly without filtration into the main; and as the waters from the filter beds at Lea Bridge are carried down the company's canal to two large open reservoirs of nine acres at Old Ford, the water of these reservoirs can be used, as they can at once be thrown in any quantities into the pumping wells.'* [26]

Farr's observations were supported by a further investigation undertaken in 1867 by Captain Henry Whatley Tyler for the Board of Trade. Tyler confirmed that contaminated water from the covered and uncovered reservoirs had caused the cholera outbreak.[27]

The East London Waterworks had contravened the 1852 Metropolis Water Act, which stipulated that it was unlawful to supply water for domestic use from any part of the Thames below Teddington Lock or tidal tributary rivers.[28] In addition to the negligence of the East London Water Company, Bazalgette's new northern low level sewer was not yet complete and effluent was still being discharged into the River Lea below Old Ford. Bazalgette commented:

*'It is unfortunately, just the locality where our main drainage works are not complete. The low-level sewer is constructed through the locality, but the pumping station at Abbey Mills will not be completed until next summer; therefore the drainage of the district does not yet flow into the low-level sewer. We are deodorizing the sewers and gullies freely with chloride of lime.'* [29]

It was agreed that in order to remedy the situation, a temporary pumping station should be erected at Abbey Mills, but this would take around three weeks to complete.

By the first week of August, the rate of deaths had begun to decline, yet in those seven days alone 774 had died. Farr was appalled by the number of deaths caused by the negligence at Old Ford:

*'London is divided into thirty-seven districts; six districts are supplied from Old Ford, and every one has been ravaged from the epidemic ... By the doctrines of chances, it is impossible that the coincidence between this particular water and the high mortality should be fortuitous ... during six weeks in succession.'*[30]

Whilst the water being supplied to these districts may have been tainted with sewage from further upriver, it is more likely that the contamination came from down river, as Farr realised in his consideration of the research conducted for him by the chemist Edward Frankland:

*'The bottoms of all the Old Ford reservoirs are much below the dirty sewage waters of the Lea at Trinity high-water mark; and professor Frankland shows the possibility of the accidental contamination of the waters of the covered reservoir ... This reservoir, as I was informed, is excavated in clay, but the side next to the navigation branch of the foul river Lea is of gravel.'*[31]

Conditions in the lower reaches of the Lea would have provided the ideal breeding ground for pathogenic cholera carried by the tide from the Thames Estuary. During the hot July of 1866 the brackish water was warm and rich with plankton, and just days before the epidemic escalated, would have flooded the reservoirs with contaminated water. Farr described the factors which had all combined to create the 'perfect storm' for cholera:

*'It is at Old Ford ... that the river Lea has become offensive at times, within the last few years, owing to the increase of buildings and factories within the Metropolitan area; it also has the disadvantage of being tidal below Old Ford, and therefore liable to the inflow of impurity from the Thames, and from the sewage of Stratford and West Ham, which is turned into the Bow Creek arm of the Lea without deodorization.'*[32]

Further evidence of estuary and river water contaminating the Old Ford reservoirs emerged in reports of eels and mussel shells found blocking domestic water pipes in places such as Poplar, which were supplied by The East London Water Company.

In November, as temperatures fell once again, cholera was on the wane but there was a sudden outbreak in Woolwich following heavy rainfall and flooding. Some 73 died, causing Farr to comment:

> *'The great outfall sewer has probably had little effect on the outbreak of cholera; but it is by no means clear that the contamination of the Thames by sewage will have no effect on the health of the people in the marshes. This must be looked to by the able engineers of the Metropolitan Board.'* [33]

According to Farr's report, by the end of the 1866 outbreak there had been 14,378 registered deaths from cholera and 17,170 from diarrhoea in England. London registered deaths from cholera amounted to 5,596 and from diarrhoea 3,147, and of these in the East End (comprising the districts of Shoreditch, Bethnal Green, Whitechapel, St George-in-the-East, Stepney, Mile End Old Town, and Poplar) registered deaths from cholera and diarrhoea were approximately 3,941 and 909 respectively.[34]

Farr's investigations and his 1866 report showed that, above all else, the polluted waters of the Lea and Thames were the cause of the East End cholera outbreak. Yet Farr realised, as his biographer, John M. Eyler, underlines, that the outbreak was a 'complex socio-medical phenomenon.'[35] However, this did not alter the trust Farr had in statistics. According to Eyler, 'He retained a belief in the power of numerical empiricism to cut through the apparent complexity of socio-medical phenomena to discover fundamental laws governing human existence.'[36] Farr's use of statistics and his methodology were powerful and won over those who had not been convinced by Snow's work, which they believed was insufficiently backed up by numerical data. Later, in 1870, in his *Twelfth Annual Report of the Medical Officer to the Privy Council*, Dr John Simon declared his support for the waterborne theory and lamented the conclusions of the 1854 Committee for Scientific Enquiries.[37]

However, before this admission and in the midst of the cholera outbreak, Simon already understood there was a need to reform sanitation and living conditions and he was instrumental in the passing of the 1866 Sanitary Act – a landmark in the history of public health and, indeed, in his own career. On 11 August, *The Times* reported its opinion of the legislation:

> '*The "Sanitary Act, 1866," then, does, for the first time in our history, put the public health upon the ground on which it ought to stand, enforcing the local authorities to it ... and it introduces ... a new sanitary era. Great honour is due to Mr. Simon, to whose unwearied zeal, ability and public spirit was are indebted.*'[38]

At the height of the cholera outbreak, the new Sanitary Act put the responsibility for every aspect of the supply of pure water and sewage management in the control of local authorities, including provision and maintenance. The Act also amended the existing Nuisances Removal Acts and gave local authorities better defined powers to deal with related matters such as rubbish and pollution, domestic overcrowding, workplace conditions and the state of lodging houses.

The Act addressed the role of local authorities in the face of outbreaks of infectious disease, such as cholera, and contained elements similar to those Budd and Davies had put in place in Bristol. It required the provision of free disinfection and the carriage of the sick to a hospital; it gave doctors the right to remove the infectious dead and to take the sick to a hospital; it also enforced the provision of places for the dead. The Act required local authorities to be aware of infection, in order to prevent items such as soiled bedding being sold on, for instance, and to understand the importance of disinfection in areas previously inhabited by the sick. Moreover, there was provision for complaint should sewers be in a poor state of repair, a clause which provided a 'mode of proceeding where [a] sewer authority has made default.'[39]

Further changes came in 1871 with the formation of the Local Government Board, superseding the role of the Privy Council and bringing together staff from the Poor Law Board, General Register Office, and the Local Government Act Office. Public Health Acts in 1872 and 1875 continued sanitation reform with an emphasis on local responsibility.[40] The 1875 Act tightened controls on sanitation and building, and addressed urban infrastructure, such as roads. It also created port sanitary authorities and consolidated a considerable amount of earlier legislation, including the 1874 Sanitary Laws Amendment Act and the 1847 Town Improvement Clauses Act, although none of this applied to Scotland, Ireland or London.[41] In addition, the Artisans' Dwellings Act of 1875 gave local authorities the power to begin the process of slum clearance.

The issue of purifying sewage prior to its discharge into water courses was also addressed in the 1875 Public Health Act:

> ' ... this Act shall authorise any local authority to make or use any sewer drain or outfall for the purpose of conveying sewage or filthy water into any natural stream or water course, or into any canal pond or lake until such sewage or filthy water is freed from all excrementitious or other foul or noxious matter such as would affect or deteriorate the purity and quality of the water.'[42]

The 1866 outbreak of cholera in Woolwich had shown that those areas close to the outfalls of Bazalgette's new system were now vulnerable to waterborne diseases such as cholera and typhoid. In the summer of 1877 the Thames Conservancy instructed Captain Edward Killwick Calver, R.N., and Doctors Letheby and Williamson to examine the soil of the river bed close to the outfalls and at Woolwich Reach. Concern had been raised because of sediment levels causing a problem for shipping and a decrease in levels of fish such as whitebait and shrimps. Their conclusions criticised Bazalgette's scheme and his calculations of how sewage would be discharged and move seaward. The recommendation was that the Metropolitan Board of Works should dredge the river,[43] but Bazalgette did not take the criticism lightly and a dispute ensued.

The following summer a paddle steamer, *The Princess Alice*, collided with *The Bywell Castle*, a steam collier, in the Thames Estuary, killing over 570 people. The aftermath of the accident confirmed fears that the lower reaches of the river were dangerously polluted. However, as sanitary historian Stephen Halliday has observed, the incident, 'sharpened the dispute but did little to resolve it.'[44]

Days out were becoming increasingly affordable for Londoners in the late nineteenth century, and the two shilling return trip to the Rosherville Gardens in Gravesend was one of the most popular. *The Princess Alice* was a large saloon steamer, licensed to carry over 800 pleasure-seekers. On 3 September 1878, she left Sheerness at 4.15 pm, docking at Gravesend at 6.30 pm, to pick up passengers at the Gardens. The weather had been particularly warm and, as the day trippers crowded onto the decks, the steamer set off on her voyage up river to the North Woolwich pier; on board were 228 men, 340 women and about 145 children.[45]

Around an hour later, at Barking Reach the vessel was progressing at a rate of around 11 knots an hour. The crew perceived the lights of the *Bywell Castle* ahead, travelling at about 5.5 knots as she rounded Bull's Point and entered the Reach. Suddenly the steam collier was upon the *Princess Alice* and in the confusion the crew was ordered to put her helm to starboard, rather than to port, as is the rule for passing vessels. The massive steam collier slammed into the *Princess Alice*, penetrating her side to a depth of some 14 feet, engulfing the engine room with water and causing the middle section to sink.

Within just five minutes, the *Princess Alice* had split in half and most of the passengers, including whole families, had perished. Charles and Elizabeth Teesdale from Bridge Street in Westminster, a young couple in their twenties, died with their children Elizabeth, aged seven, Joseph, aged 15 months, and Charles's nine-year-old sister, Amelia. Zinc plate worker John Anckorn, aged 49, from Waterloo Place in Southwark and his 47-year-old wife, Ellen, were both killed and left behind seven orphaned children. Also dead was a 24-year-old publisher's clerk named Benjamin Baker from Camberwell, who had recently been married.[46]

Their bodies were taken to the dockyard at Woolwich, the only place nearby that was large enough to house the hundreds of bodies lifted from the Thames. Many of the victims could only be identified by their clothing or the colour of their hair, such was the toxic effect of the polluted water. Many of the drowned were never identified and of an estimated 115 recorded missing,[47] some were never found.

On Friday, 27 September the Metropolitan Board of Works held its first meeting following the disaster. The next day, *The Times* reported the committee's discussion of the sinking of the *Princess Alice*, in which Board member Mr Richardson described the water of the River Thames as 'poisonous ... its taste and smell something it was impossible to describe.'[48] The committee had also questioned 'whether such state of the water ... arose from the main drainage outfalls.'[49]

Reports in the press confirmed that most of the passengers had drowned, however, the Registrar's Returns published in December in *The Times* disclosed that: 'In addition to these 574 deaths from drowning several deaths of persons on board the *Princess Alice* have been registered which were directly referred to the immersion ... not caused by drowning.'[50] Articles were already being published in the newspapers suggesting that, in the aftermath, some of the survivors and those trapped on board the vessel had died from ingesting polluted river water.

In the weeks prior to the *Princess Alice* disaster, statistics published in *The Times* confirmed that diarrhoea and 'simple' cholera had been the cause of some 1,592 fatalities[51] and most of those who died were, once again, from East London. Effluent from this part of the capital would have emptied into the Thames Estuary from the sewage outlets at Barking and Crossness, close by to where the *Princess Alice* sank. Contemporary reports and analysts, such as a Mr Wigner appointed by the Woolwich Board of Health,[21] described pollutants in the water such as ammonia, chloride of sodium and sulphuric acid.[53]

In a paper entitled, 'Thames Water, its Impurities, Dangers and Contaminations', Mr H. C. Burdett commented that the state of the river 'added materially to the horrors of one of the most terrible calamities which has occurred in modern times.'[54] Indeed, the river was polluted to such an extent that sewage and slime had weighed down the bulky clothing of the female victims and impeded any attempt they could have made to save themselves. Such was the case of Mrs F. Marshall of Deptford, who had died because her husband could no longer support her weight as they attempted to swim to safety.[55] Burdett described 'a vast mass of polluted water, eight miles long, 750 yards wide and 4½ ft. in depth, charged with offensive matter, both fluid and solid,' which was carried up to four times daily back and forth by the tidal waters of the Thames between Gravesend and Blackwall. Other reports concluded that this mass must have contained around 21 days' build-up of sewage.[56]

Such conclusions began to cast a shadow over Bazalgette's sewage system and representatives of the Metropolitan Board of Works, including Bazalgette himself, began an examination of the waters of the Thames, taking samples from various locations. They paid particular attention to the stretches that appeared most polluted, and especially the area where the *Princess Alice* sank. Their initial conclusions gave no reason for alarm, as the analysis of the river water was based on no more than a visual interpretation. Bazalgette reiterated the comments he had directed to Captain Calver's investigation the previous year, that the mud banks on the river were 'not formed of sewage, but of natural deposits.'[57] The Board concluded that the *Princess Alice* had stirred up poisons from the depths of an otherwise untainted river.[58]

In November 1878, Mr Kimber from the Plumstead District Board of Works observed that whilst the 1865 Act of Parliament had recommended the transportation of sewage some 24 miles below Barking Creek, this had still not been achieved, because the company undertaking the task for the Metropolitan Board of Works had collapsed. Kimber's view was that the problem had been swept under the carpet and, as long as sewage was no longer polluting the centre of London, the Metropolitan Board of Works remained unconcerned.[59]

A review in 1880 concluded that river navigation had improved since the outfalls had been built, yet subsequently pressure grew and two years later a Royal Commission on Metropolitan Sewage Discharge was appointed. Eventually, after many years and much discussion, a solution was reached whereby precipitating channels were constructed at Barking and Crossness from which sludge would then be dumped at sea. The first vessel to begin this process in 1887 was named the *Bazalgette*.[60]

# CHAPTER 10

# A Modern Disease: Genetics, vaccines and the new theories

Following the 1866 outbreak in the East End of London, epidemic cholera was never again to occur in Britain. The pandemic of 1863, which caused so many deaths, took nine years to reach its conclusion.[1] A fifth pandemic began in 1881 and by 1892, when cholera began to rage in Hamburg, there was considerable concern that ships would bring the disease across the North Sea to England. In the end, around 135 deaths in Britain were attributed to cholera in 1892. The victims had all recently arrived from abroad[2] but each outbreak was confined, and the disease remained at bay. Then, in 1899, with the emergence of the sixth pandemic, whilst cholera broke out in Southern Europe[3] Britain was spared once again.

During the outbreak in Calcutta in 1884, German scientist Robert Koch finally identified the cholera bacterium, *Vibrio cholerae*, paving the way for the future of epidemiology. Koch proved that cholera was caused by a micro-organism and the arguments against it being a waterborne disease became more fragile, though many, including miasmatist Florence Nightingale, remained unconvinced. Work continued in the fight against cholera, with the development of a vaccine in the 1890s by Waldemar Mordecai Wolff-Hakine at the Pasteur Institute in Paris.[4]

In recent years more work has been done to improve cholera vaccines, targeting the intestinal tract, where an immune response would be most effective. A prototype vaccine was developed in Sweden in the 1980s by Professor Jan Holmgren, whose new oral vaccine not only contained killed cholera cells (as the earlier vaccines had done) but also a protein subunit of the cholera toxin, known as the B subunit. Trials led by Professor Dr John Clemens began in Bangladesh in 1983 with a group of 90,000 people, including children. The trials proved successful and the vaccine, known as Dukoral, was approved by the World Health Organisation (WHO).

The use of Dukoral on a wider scale was to prove costly, however, particularly as it required refrigeration and mixing with a buffer solution of sodium hydrogen carbonate before oral ingestion. Holmgren and Clemens were involved with further research in Vietnam and when the International Vaccine Institute was founded in South Korea in the 1990s, work began to move on apace, particularly as a result of further financial support from benefactors, including the Bill and Melinda Gates Foundation. A more affordable two-dose oral vaccine (measuring less than half a teaspoon) was developed, containing whole cholera cells, which was licensed in India by the name of Shanchol. This vaccine was later discovered to increase levels of herd immunity, whereby those who have received the vaccine prevent the spread of the disease to others in their community.[5]

The introduction of the vaccine was overseen in Bangladesh by the International Centre for Diarrhoeal Disease Research (ICDDR,B). The vaccine was shown to be effective when used in areas and groups with a high cholera risk and it has subsequently been used in Guinea, Zanzibar, Mozambique, Haiti and on refugees in South Sudan. Since the successful introduction of this preventative measure, humanitarian organisations around the world have come together to promote the safe and more widespread use of the vaccine in countries where cholera is a threat to public health.

One such group, DOVE (Delivering Oral Vaccine Efficiently), based at John Hopkins University in the United States, has been working with WHO and UNICEF. DOVE's slogan for cholera prevention is, 'STOP Cholera: Work Together. Stop Transmission,'[6] Slogans such as this are important tools for humanitarian organisations, as one of their greatest obstacles is complacency and they need to ensure that communities under threat of cholera understand that a vaccine is not a miracle cure. Preventative medicine will only work effectively where attention is also paid to good sanitation. Director of DOVE, epidemiologist, Professor David A. Sack, MD, explains:

> '[Cholera vaccine] *is not at all a replacement for water/sanitation, and in fact, the vaccine and sanitation should be synergistic. If one had better hygiene, the 'dose' of vibrios people are exposed to would be reduced – this makes the vaccine more effective. And if people were vaccinated, they would excrete fewer bacteria into the environment, making the water sanitation program more effective.'*[7]

The development and employment of more effective vaccines is as a result of an even more advanced understanding of the structure of the micro-organisms that cause disease, and the genetic sequencing of *Vibrio cholerae* has also made it possible to compose a 'cholera family tree', demonstrating how recent epidemics are related to each other. The Wellcome Trust Sanger Institute in Cambridge is at the forefront of this work, and here Professor Nicholas Thomson employs 'genomic techniques to understand infectious disease in the context of global health.'[8] Thomson explains:

> '*Essentially we are defining the global population structure of the current pandemic wave of cholera known as Pandemic 7 El Tor ... Using the genome sequence to plot the ancestry of isolates causing outbreaks today and over the last 50 or so years. Through this analysis we can determine what has happened to cholera over that time and how the different isolates collected from human cholera cases are related to each other all over the world. This work showed that actually the isolates causing the majority of the disease in the world currently are related to each other and have only diverged from an ancestral strain recently before spreading in three independent waves globally.*
> '*Interestingly by combining the phylogenetic* [evolutionary relationship] *data with the dates and place*

*of isolation we were able to show that the ancestor of all three global waves of Pandemic 7 El Tor cholera emerged from the Bay of Bengal and radiated out from there. So just like John Snow looking in London we identified our global pump. Of course mirroring John Snow we now need to figure how to take the handle off that pump.'[9]*

Even in the twenty-first century, cholera is still a significant threat to public health, infecting some three to five million people a year and resulting in between 100,000 to 200,000 deaths.[10] Recent outbreaks have affected Latin and South America, Mexico, Africa, Indonesia, India, Bangladesh, and Haiti.

As discussed in Chapter 1, cholera can be divided into two types, or serogroups. The pathogenic O1 type, known as Classical Cholera, was responsible for pandemics one to six, which began in 1817, 1826, 1852, 1863, 1881 and 1899. The seventh and current pandemic is caused by the O139 serogroup, known as El Tor (as explained above by Thomson) and emerged in 1961 in Sulawesi, Indonesia. Work by Sandra Moore, Nicholas Thomson et al. has revealed that:

*' ... each successive wave of disease since that initial outbreak originated from a single clone, very distinct from the classical strains of the previous pandemic ... analysis of the seventh pandemic strains also shows that V. cholerae has continually evolved in South Asia and spread around the globe in at least three independent but overlapping waves. The three waves share a common ancestor dating back to the 1950s.'[11]*

Cholera's pathogenic types or serogroups acquire their toxicity through horizontal gene transfer with bacteriophages, a type of virus, common in the natural environment such as estuaries and coastal areas. Cholera pandemics comprise waves of disease which may be genetically distinct. Work at Sanger has shown that the first wave of El Tor was different because it acquired an additional gene during the horizontal gene transfer process. This gene increased the efficiency by which the cholera vibrio or bacterium could produce toxin. Cholera bacteria which caused the second and third waves of Pandemic 7 subsequently acquired additional elements which encode resistance to antibiotics. This, and the adaptation to produce the pathogenic toxin more efficiently, means that later strains of cholera in Pandemic 7 spread more rapidly from person to person and produced more severe symptoms.[12]

Further research conducted on cholera at Sanger has sequenced the genomes of 154 strains of *Vibrio cholerae*, and this has revealed that antibiotic resistance was acquired in about 1982, just as the second wave of Pandemic 7 emerged.

Today cholera is treated with oral and intravenous rehydration, and occasionally by antibiotics. It is exposure to these antibiotics which enabled the Pandemic 7 strains of cholera to acquire resistance, and this has affected the way in which the disease has subsequently spread around the globe throughout Africa, Asia, Europe and the Americas. However, using genetic identification scientists such as those at Sanger, have been able to track cholera and their research has shown that the disease is spread by human movement, rather than evolving from local strains of non-pathogenic *Vibrio cholerae*.

In 2011 Professor Gordon Dougan, Sanger's Head of Pathogen Research, commented: 'We regard the Bay of Bengal as the ultimate source of *V. cholerae*. The strains can then evolve further outside this region, but they eventually die out and are replaced by the next sweep from the Bay.'[13]

Research has also revealed that the current strains of pathogenic cholera are subsets of clones and not a diverse range of evolved, environmental strains;[14] they are branches of the same cholera family tree. Moreover, as Dougan explained, cholera evolves in India's Bay of Bengal and successive waves are then spread to the rest of the world by the movement of people, just as it did on board ships crossing the seas in the nineteenth century. Cholera epidemics break out in areas where the disease has not previously been known and where there is little resistance, which, again, is what happened in the 1800s, when cholera broke out in countries where it was previously unknown.

A paper published in *Nature* in 2011 presented some of the

conclusions of the research conducted at Sanger supporting the view that all cholera outbreaks since the 1950s have their origin in a common Indian ancestor:

*'Despite clear evidence of sporadic long-range transmission events that are likely to be associated with direct human carriage, the overall pattern seen in our data is one of continued local evolution of* V. cholerae *in the Bay of Bengal, with several independent waves of global transmission resulting in short-term epidemics in non-endemic countries.'* [15]

With communication between countries becoming ever faster and more frequent, successive waves of cholera will continue to emerge from India and spread across the world. Air travel facilitates that rapid spread and areas of the globe that have never experienced cholera become more vulnerable, particularly as indigenous communities have little resistance to unknown diseases. Vulnerability is enhanced during natural disasters, when aid workers carrying infections arrive to help an already weakened population. This was what happened in Haiti when, in January 2010, the country was hit by an earthquake measuring over 7 on the Richter scale. Thousands were killed, but it was the displacement of around a quarter of a million people that would provide the opportunity for cholera to break out. The epidemic continues to be a major public health issue and by the end of 2014 it had spread to nine of Haiti's ten regional departments. Between 2010 and 2015, almost 9,000 people in Haiti have died from cholera,[16] and it is now widely agreed that the disease was brought to the country by UN workers from Nepal, where cholera is endemic.

The situation in Haiti provided an opportunity to observe epidemic cholera in a similar way as Dr John Snow did in London in 1854. Then contagionists and anti-contagionists put forward their views, and in Haiti a similar argument has ensued as two camps have emerged: those who believe cholera was an imported toxic strain, as discussed above, and those who believe that cholera arose from the natural environment.

A MODERN DISEASE

Epidemiologist and historian Dr Ralph Frerichs has documented the life and work of Snow on his website,[17] which is hosted by the Department of Epidemiology at the University of California, and also includes information on other epidemic diseases. Aware of the similar opportunity Haiti has given for research, Frerichs has taken a keen interest in the outbreak and the arguments which have emerged; here he gives the background:

'With the two theories in mind, epidemiological detective work was soon under way. The Haitian government asked the French Embassy to secure the services of French epidemiologist Renaud Piarroux, which they did. Piarroux arrived in Port-au-Prince two weeks after the epidemic was first reported, and stayed for three weeks to complete his extensive investigation. Even earlier, enterprising journalists heard rumors that cholera might have been brought by Nepalese replacement troops to a United Nations peacekeeping camp deep in the interior of the country. The camp lies near the town of Mirebalais, but has passing streams that enter the large Artibonite River that flows from the Dominican Republic border to the Caribbean Sea. One of the journalists wrote that cholera was evident in Nepal before the troops left home; the Nepalese replacement troops had arrived shortly before the epidemic onset in three shifts on October 9, 12 and 16; and their destination camp near Mirebalais had many sanitation problems.

'Piarroux's epidemiological investigation found this and much more. Early cholera cases had occurred near the Nepalese camp, followed in a few days by an enormous wave of new cases in communities near the lower Artibonite River, suggesting cholera arrived with the river flow. These cases generated new cases and gradually, the disease spread throughout the country. Piarroux's was especially convincing with his use of maps, identifying new cholera cases over time in the 140 communes that

197

*comprise the country. He was able to show where cholera started, how it quickly spread in down river communities, and then moved out to the remaining country.*

*'Other scientists studied the newly arrived* Vibrio cholerae *organism in Haiti. They found that the microbe came from a single strain and arrived in Haiti as a single event, different than would have been expected if evolving from the environment. Later when the outbreak-causing organism had an opportunity to further change, scientists measured the rate of evolution and then looked back in time. Using a molecular clock model they estimated that the organism arrived in Haiti in 2010 between July 23 and October 17, the span that includes the arrival of the replacement troops from Nepal.*

*'Perhaps the strongest laboratory information came from a study of cholera isolates collected in Nepal prior to the troops leaving for Haiti compared with cholera specimens gathered during the early phases of the epidemic in Haiti. Using a powerful new tool − whole-genome sequence typing (WGST) − the investigators found three Nepalese isolates that were nearly identical to the organism in Haiti. By "nearly," the difference was a mere 1- or 2-base pairs (i.e., the building blocks of the microbe's DNA double helix), out of a total of over four million base-pairs reported in the* Vibrio cholerae *genome.*

*With such overwhelming evidence, the tide of scientific opinion changed, accepting a story-line that originally started with rumors, proceeded with observations of journalists, and ended with the epidemiological investigations of Renaud Piarroux and the studies of many laboratory scientists. The story had its beginning in far away Nepal, a developing country as poor as Haiti.*

*'Before leaving Nepal, peacekeepers were not tested for cholera, even though cholera was present in the country. When they arrived in Haiti, there was no independent assessment of their health status. Shortly after the*

*replacement troops appeared, the epidemic started in two clusters of Haitian cases. The first cluster – much smaller in size – occurred from October 16 to 19, with all cases remaining in the Mirebalais region. The index cases, while never identified, most likely came from the Nepalese peacekeeping camp.*

*'The second cluster – now much larger in size – occurred in the lower Artibonite River region on October 19-20 where contamination of the seven communes in the river valley occurred simultaneously. The spread of cholera was statistically linked to the Artibonite River. The number of new cases and deaths dropped dramatically after only two days, suggesting a rapid decrease in cholera contamination in the passing river.*

*'On further investigation, it appears that once cholera cases accumulated in the Nepalese camp near Mirebalais, a sanitation company commissioned by the United Nations, picked up the camp sewage and, allegedly, rather than driving back to Port-au-Prince, dumped the contents into the river. The cholera-laden sewage formed a plume that flowed during the night from the camp to the Artibonite River and then by morning to the downriver communities, initiating a series of point-source outbreaks as the river flowed by. Thereafter, human activity further spread cholera throughout the country, resulting in a great epidemic.*

*'Once Piarroux and his colleagues understood how the epidemic had originated, they proceeded to plan their intervention, similar to what occurred years earlier in the island nation of Madagascar. The country had been free of cholera for decades. Then in 1999 the disease first emerged in a harbor city, probably coming by maritime transport from the nearby Comoros where cholera was present. For three years, cholera raged in Madagascar, but then quickly died out, with only a handful of cases in 2002 and 2003, and then none thereafter. The local*

199

*officials had a system in place to report suspicious cases and deaths. They treated the cases, including intravenous rehydration, educated the public and disinfected the houses. Mass immunization was not employed at the time due to the considerable expense. Cholera was eliminated and has officially remained eliminated.*

*'The same thing is being tried in Haiti. With the help of UNICEF, local public health workers have been looking for cholera during the dry season when fewer cases occur, using a commune-specific surveillance system to identify and target active foci of the disease. Once case-transmission is diminished – as verified by microbiological testing – control actions are immediately started to provide access to clean water and free distribution of treatment products, including oral rehydration kits and antibiotics where appropriate.'*[18]

Like researchers at Sanger and others around the world, Frerichs is of the opinion that 'human-activity explains the origin and transmission, not the ever-present environment,' and that the DNA evidence cannot be ignored.

The second camp of scientists believe that cholera arose from the natural environment and that the situation is more complex. In the United States Professor Rita Colwell presented her view that cholera 'needs to be redefined' and that it 'represents several infectious diseases' in an April 2014 speech to the Society for General Microbiology.[19]

Colwell's research in Haiti, with Dr Anwar Huq in Bangladesh at the ICDDR,B and at universities in America, England and France, has revealed a much closer relationship between cholera and the environment than was previously thought. The life cycle of *Vibrio cholerae* is dependent on rainfall, flooding and the depth of rivers, sea surface temperatures, salinity, and most critical of all, plankton, (as discussed in Chapter 1).

Work conducted by Colwell with the team at the ICDDR,B has shown that the pathogenicity of cholera is determined by a variety of factors and that the disease should be defined as two separate diseases:

*endemic* and *epidemic*. Colwell's new definition of cholera explains many of the observations in the nineteenth century, including why mortality was consistently higher in low-lying estuarine areas, and also in places such as Bilston in 1832 and Mecca in 1865, where population density was increased due to a large influx of people from outside.

Colwell has shown that *endemic* cholera outbreaks occur only on the coast. These are affected by environmental conditions, occurring with rises in sea surface temperatures, heights, and chlorophyll levels – all of which have an impact on plankton populations, the food source for the cholera bacterium. Satellite imagery is able to monitor these levels and for many years, (with only one exception in 1998 when monsoon rains arrived later than usual), cholera outbreaks have been accurately predicted. On the other hand, *epidemic* cholera only occurs inland. These outbreaks follow a combination of events, including above average temperatures for two months or more, intense rainfall, and a dense gathering of people, coupled with insanitary conditions.

In Haiti Colwell's researchers observed a similar dichotomy, believing the incidences of cholera on the Artibonite River and the coast represent two separate outbreaks. An analysis of the river flow indicated to them that cholera could not have been brought to the coast in this way, but the natural disaster combined with record high air temperatures and rainfall all came together at the same time to create what Colwell calls 'a perfect storm for cholera.'[20]

The situation in Haiti has a correlation with London's 1866 outbreak when cholera devastated the East End, which was meticulously observed by William Farr. He also observed the same environmental changes as Colwell, including the correlation between mortality and elevation, but he did not have the means to form a conclusion. The first outbreak of cholera occurred in the summer of 1866, when the Old Ford reservoirs were contaminated by water containing cholera from the River Lea and the Thames Estuary. Then, as mortality began to decrease and temperatures cooled, there was a second violent outbreak in November in Woolwich close to the coast following heavy rainfall and flooding. Colwell's work suggests that the inland 1866 East End outbreak was *epidemic* and the coastal Woolwich outbreak was *endemic*.

Colwell's team has also looked at *Vibrio cholerae* DNA, using a method so precise that it can discern both bacterial species and strains. In other words, it can differentiate between the pathogenic O1 and O139 strains of the bacterium, which may have been brought in from outside, and the non pathogenic non-O1/O139 types of cholera – free swimming vibrios – which may already be present in local water systems. As other researchers had shown, the faeces of cholera victims in Haiti contained *Vibrio cholerae* O1, the pathogenic strain which causes the disease and the genetic composition of which resembles 'concurrent epidemic isolates from South Asia and Africa.'[21] But Colwell's work showed that the faeces of Haiti's cholera victims also contained the non pathogenic '*V. cholerae* non-O1/O139 populations [which] were not clonal but most probably serve as a reservoir for genomic and pathogenicity islands.'[22] Colwell's conclusion was that if both strains are present in the faeces of cholera victims then there must be a relationship between the different cholera strains. Colwell noted that the genetic similarity of the pathogenic and non pathogenic strains would make this possible: '*V. cholerae* non-O1/O139 populations ... harbor a genomic backbone similar to that of toxigenic *V. cholerae* O1 circulating in the Western hemisphere.'[23]

If Colwell and her team are correct, then their hypothesis may begin to explain the reasons behind the way in which cholera spread through the British Isles in the nineteenth century. Those living in estuarine and coastal areas were worse affected than others and cholera spread along the waterways and the coast from the mouths of rivers, where cholera had been deposited from the effluent of victims arriving by ship from areas where pathogenic cholera was already prevalent. Then, not only was cholera carried by humans, by boat and on goods from one place to another, but benign free swimming cholera bacteria in the estuaries, rivers and canals were interacting with external pathogenic strains introduced by boats and ships to create a more toxic form of the disease.

Colwell's work in India has also shown that there is a relationship between *Vibrio cholerae* and other intestinal pathogens, though this is complex and not yet fully understood. However, it seems to indicate that different populations, including those in the West, have a greater or lesser tolerance to gastric infections, depending on intestinal bacterial flora. The implications of this for Colwell's work and for understanding cholera outbreaks is that there may be a relationship between pathogenic and non-pathogenic micro-organisms within the intestinal tract.[24]

The work on the genome sequencing of cholera by teams such as those at the Sanger Institute in Cambridge, has shown that the pathogenic cholera bacterium is clonal and successive waves of the disease will continue to surge out from the Bay of Bengal, seizing on opportunities such as natural disasters and breaking out at epidemic levels. However, if Professor Rita Colwell's hypothesis is correct and the endemic cholera outbreaks which occur in coastal and estuarine regions are intrinsically linked to the environment, it may be impossible to ever eradicate cholera. If global warming brings a rise in sea levels and temperatures then these outbreaks – and their intensity – will increase.

In 1854 when cholera violently broke out in London's Soho, Dr John Snow was able to convince the Board of Guardians of St James's Parish to remove the handle of the pump in Broad Street. Today cholera is still a threat to public health across the world, killing up to 200,000 each year, but we cannot remove a pump handle to prevent this continuing. Moreover, with the possibility that there may be an environmental factor at work in the development of pathogenic cholera, perhaps the wrong water pump has been identified, and if this is the case, then we run the risk of removing the wrong handle.

Cholera was the plague of the Victorian era but there is every possibility that, given the right circumstances, cholera – and Colwell's 'perfect storm' – could make an unwelcome return in the twenty-first century.

# Notes

**Introduction**
1. McMaster University, *Daily News*, (27 January 2014), 'Scientists Reveal Cause of one of the most Devastating Pandemics in Human History,' *Daily News*, http://dailynews.mcmaster.ca [2014].
2. Barney Sloane, *The Black Death in London*, (Stroud: The History Press, 2011), p.83.
3. 'London Plagues 1348-1665,' www.museumoflondon.org.uk/files/5613/7053/1233/London_plagues_13481665.pdf [2014].
4. Bos et al, 'A draft genome of Yersinia pestis from victims of the Black Death,' pp.506–510.
5. Ibid.
6. Ian Kershaw, 'The Great Famine And Agrarian Crisis In England 1315-1322,' *Past and Present*, 59(1), http://links.jstor.org [2014].
7. Daniel Defoe, *A Journal of the Plague Year*, (London: George Routledge and Sons, 1886), pp.249-250.
8. John Richetti: *The Life of Daniel Defoe: A Critical Biography*, (Wiley-Blackwell, 2008), p.308.
9. B.S. Drasar, B.D. Forrest, *Cholera and the Ecology of* Vibrio cholerae, (Springer,1996).
10. 'The Year Without a Summer,' www.bellrock.org.uk/misc/misc_year.htm [2014].
11. *The Times*, 20 October 1847.
12. John Glyde, *The Moral, Social and Religious Condition of Ipswich in the Middle of the Nineteenth Century*, (Ipswich: J.M. Burton & Co,1850; BiblioLife, 2009).
13. William Budd, 'Asiatic Cholera in Bristol in 1866,' (*British Medical Journal*, 13 April 1867; v. 1(328), MCID: PMC2309505); www.ncbi.nlm.nih.gov/pmc/articles/PMC2309505
14. Ibid.

**Chapter 1 An Ancient Disease**
1. B.S. Drasar, B.D. Forrest, *Cholera and the Ecology of* Vibrio cholerae, (Springer,1996), p.19.
2. John Bell, David Francis Condie, *All the Material Facts in the History of Epidemic Cholera* etc., (Philadelphia: Thomas Desilver, 1832), p.143.
3. Thomas Sydenham, *The Works of Thomas Sydenham, M.D., on Acute and Chronic Diseases: With Their Histories and Modes of Cure*, (Philadelphia B. & T. Kite, 1809), p.103.
4. Ibid, p. 106.
5. J. N. Hays, *Epidemics and Pandemics: Their Impacts on Human History*, (Santa Barbara, California: ABC-CLIO, 2005), p.197.
6. Romesh Chunder Dutt, *The Economic History of India in the Victorian Age: From the Accession of Queen Victoria in 1837 to the Commencement of the Twentieth Century*, (London: Routledge, 2013), pp.166-178.

# NOTES

7. M. Durey, *The First Spasmodic Cholera Epidemic in York, 1832* (York: St Anthony's Press, 1974), p.2.

8. James Johnson, *The Medico-Chirurgical Review and Journal of Practical Medicine* Vol. 20, (S. Highley, 1832), p.266.

9. Ibid, p. 297.

10. *The Quarterly Review,* Vol. XLVI, November 1831 and January 1832, (London: John Murray, 1832).

11. Michael Dunnill, *Dr William Budd, Bristol's most famous physician,* (Bristol: Redcliffe, 2006), p.35.

12. Christopher Hamlin, *Cholera: The Biography,* (Oxford University Press, 2009), p. 23.

13. James Johnson, *The Medico-Chirurgical Review and Journal of Practical Medicine* Vol. 20, (S. Highley, 1832), p.283.

14. François Gabriel Boisseau, *A Treatise on Cholera Morbus: Or, Researches on the Symptoms, Nature, and Treatment of the Disease: And on the Different Means of Avoiding it,* (New York: Collins & Co, 1832).

15. David Gladstone, and Samuel Edward Finer, *Edwin Chadwick: Nineteenth-century Social Reform,* (London: Routledge, 1997), p.342.

16. John M. Eyler, 'William Farr on the Cholera: The Sanitarian's Disease Theory and the Statistician's Method,' p.82.

17. Ibid.

18. Ibid , pp.82-3.

19. James Johnson, *The Medico-Chirurgical Review and Journal of Practical Medicine,* Vol. 20, (S. Highley, 1832), p.276.

20. Klose K.E., Mekalanos J.J., (1998), 'Distinct roles of an alternative sigma factor during both free-swimming and colonizing phases of the Vibrio cholerae pathogenic cycle,' *Molecular Microbiology,* 28(3), pp.501-20, www.ncbi.nlm.nih.gov/pubmed/9632254 [2014].

21. Dr Rita Colwell, 'Climate Change, Oceans and Infectious Disease: Cholera Pandemics as a Model,' Annual Conference of the Society of General Microbiology, April 2014.

22. *The Times*, 10 August 1866.

23. World Health Organization, (2003), 'Algae and cyanobacteria in coastal and estuarine waters,' *Guidelines For Safe Recreational Water Environments, Volume 1: Coastal And Fresh Waters;* Chapter 7, www.who.int/water_sanitation_health/bathing/srwe1-chap7.pdf [2014].

24. Ibid.

25 Glenn Rhodes et al, (2014), '*Mycobacterium avium* Subspecies *paratuberculosis*: Human Exposure through Environmental and Domestic Aerosols,' *Pathogens,* 3(3), pp.577, www.mdpi.com/2076-0817/3/3/577 [2014].

26. M. Elias Dueker, Gregory D. O'Mullan, 'Aeration remediation of a polluted waterway increases near-surface coarse and culturable microbial aerosols,' (*Science of the Total Environment,* 478, 2014), pp.184-9.

27. Glenn Rhodes et al, (2014), '*Mycobacterium avium* Subspecies *paratuberculosis*: Human Exposure through Environmental and Domestic Aerosols,' *Pathogens,* 3(3), pp.577-95, www.mdpi.com/2076-0817/3/3/577 [2014].

28. Professor Roger Pickup, Division of Biomedical and Life Sciences, Lancaster University, 17 October 2014 (unpublished).

29. Ronald G. Labbé, Santos García, *Guide to Foodborne Pathogens*, (Chichester: Wiley-Blackwell, 2013).
30. David A. Sack, R. Bradley Sack, G. Balakrish Nair, and A. K. Siddique, 'Cholera,' (*The Lancet*, Vol. 363 (17 January 2004), www.ph.ucla.edu/epi/snow/lancet363_223_233_2004.pdf, p.229, [2014].
31. Shah M. Faruque, G. Balakrish Nair, *Vibrio Cholerae: Genomics and Molecular Biology*, (Horizon Scientific Press, 2008), p.86.
32. B.J. Haley et al., 'Genomic and Phenotypic Characterization of *Vibrio cholerae* Non-O1 Isolates from a US Gulf Coast Cholera Outbreak,' *PLoS One*, 9(4), www.ncbi.nlm.nih.gov/pubmed/24699521 [2014].
33. Shah, MA et al., (2014), 'Genomic epidemiology of Vibrio cholerae O1 associated with floods, Pakistan, 2010,' Emerging Infectious Diseases Journal, 20 (1), http://dx.doi.org/10.3201/eid2001.130428 [2014].
34. Melanie Blokesch, 'The Lifestyle of *Vibrio cholerae* Fosters Gene Transfers,' p 64.
35. Shah M. Faruque et al., 'Seasonal epidemics of cholera inversely correlate with the prevalence of environmental cholera phages,' *Proceedings of the National Academy of Sciences of the United States of America*, 102 (5), pp. 1702-7, www.ncbi.nlm.nih.gov/pubmed/15653771 [2014].
36. Dr. Rita Colwell, *Climate Change, Oceans and Infectious Disease: Cholera Pandemics as a Model*, Annual Conference of the Society of General Microbiology, April 2014.
37. Gleisel Cabuguason, 'The Microbiology of the Vibrio cholerae Bacterium,' pp.3-4
38. Princeton University, Department of Molecular Biology, Bonnie L. Bassler (http://molbio.princeton.edu/faculty/molbio-faculty/31-bassler) [2014].
39. Amanda J. Thomas, *The Lambeth Cholera Outbreak of 1848-1849: The Setting, Causes, Course and Aftermath of an Epidemic in London*, (Jefferson, North Carolina: McFarland & Co., 2009), pp.38-40; Michael L. Bennish, 'Cholera: Pathophysiology, Clinical Features and Treatment,' in I. Kaye Wachsmuth, Paul A. Blake, and Ørjan Olsvik, eds., Vibrio cholerae *and Cholera. Molecular to Global Perspectives* (Washington DC: American Society for Microbiology, 1994), pp.231-7.
40. John Hamett, 'One of the late British Medical Commission at Danzig, &c., in the North of Europe. Extracts from Medical Reports founded on actual Observation, and Communicated to the Government, on the Cholera Morbus, which Prevailed at Danzig between the end of May and First Part of September, 1831,' (*The Medico-Chirurgical Review and Journal of Practical Medicine*, Vol. 20, S. Highley, 1832), p.309.
41. Amanda J. Thomas, *The Lambeth Cholera Outbreak of 1848-1849: The Setting, Causes, Course and Aftermath of an Epidemic in London*, (Jefferson, North Carolina: McFarland & Co., 2009).
42. Ibid; E. Manby, surgeon, *Dissertation, with Practical Remarks, on Cholera Morbus*, (London: Burgess and Hill, 1831), from William Baly, *Reports on Epidemic Cholera: Drawn up at the desire of the Cholera Committee of the Royal College of Physicians*, Cholera Committee, Royal College of Physicians (London: J. Churchill, 1854), Ref. SLTr80.
43. Amanda J. Thomas, *The Lambeth Cholera Outbreak of 1848-1849: The Setting, Causes, Course and Aftermath of an Epidemic in London*, (Jefferson, North Carolina: McFarland & Co., 2009); Archibald Billing, M.D., A.M., F.R.S., 'On The Treatment of Asiatic Cholera,' 2d ed., revised (London: S. Highley, 1848), from William Baly,

# NOTES

*Reports on Epidemic Cholera: Drawn up at the desire of the Cholera Committee of the Royal College of Physicians*, Cholera Committee, Royal College of Physicians (London: J. Churchill, 1854), Ref. SLTr80.
44. World Health Organization, (www.who.int/topics/cholera/treatment/en).

## Chapter 2 Brandy is the Cure
1. James Johnson, *The Medico-Chirurgical Review and Journal of Practical Medicine* Vol. 20, (S. Highley, 1832), p.276.
2. UK Parliament Website; www.parliament.uk/about/living-heritage/transforming society/towncountry/towns/tyne-and-wear-case-study/introduction/cholera-in-sunderland [2014].
3. *The Times*, 27 October 1830.
4. *The Times*, 2 July 1831.
5. *The Times*, 18 June 1831.
6 *The Times*, 2 July 1831.
7. *The Times*, 2 July 1831.
8. *The Times*, 2 July 1831.
9 Joan Lane, *A Social History of Medicine: Health, Healing and Disease in England, 1750-1950*, (London: Routledge, 2012), p.146.
10. Arthur S. Macnalty, *British Medical Journal*, 25 September 1965, p.748.
11. John S. Morris, 'Sir Henry Halford, president of the Royal College of Physicians, with a note on his involvement in the exhumation of King Charles I,' (*Postgrad Medical Journal* 2007 June; 83(980): 431–433; www.ncbi.nlm.nih.gov/pmc/articles/PMC2600044 [2014].
12. *The Times*, 2 July 1831.
13. *The Times*, 29 July 1831.
14. *Parliamentary Papers, House of Commons and Command*, Vol. 17, (H.M. Stationery Office, 1831), p.15.
15. *The Times*, 29 July 1831.
16. *The Times*, 18 August 1831.
17. *The Edinburgh Review*, (Edinburgh, 1830), p.20.
18. *The Times*, 29 August 1831.
19. *Pigot and Co.'s National Commercial Directory of the Whole of Scotland and of The Isle of Man: with a General Alphabetical List of the Nobility, Gentry and Clergy of Scotland*, (London: James Pigot and Co, 1837).
20. Ibid.
21. *The Times*, 29 October 1831.
22. Cajeput essential oil is made from the leaves of the cajeput tree and is known for its antiseptic properties; it belongs to the to the genus *Melaleuca* and is similar to tea tree oil.
23. *The Times*, 29 October 1831.
24. Ibid.
25. James Johnson, *The Medico-Chirurgical Review and Journal of Practical Medicine* Vol. 20, (S. Highley, 1832), p.302.
26. William Reid Clanny, *Hyperanthraxis; Or, the Cholera of Sunderland*, (London: Whittaker, Treacher and Arnott, 1832), p.1.
27. Ibid.
28. Ibid, p.2; pp.8-9.

29. Victoria County History, 'How the central settlements of Sunderland grew to become a town,' *Growth of the Town, 1600-1800*, Durham Volume V: Sunderland, www.victoriacountyhistory.ac.uk/counties/durham/work-in-progress/growth-town-1600-1800 [2014].
30. William Reid Clanny, *Hyperanthraxis; Or, the Cholera of Sunderland*, (London: Whittaker, Treacher and Arnott, 1832), pp.19-20.
31. Ibid, p.20.
32. Ibid, p.19.
33. www.lancashireinfantrymuseum.org.uk/the-82nd-prince-of-waless-volunteers-regiment [2014].
34. William Reid Clanny, *Hyperanthraxis; Or, the Cholera of Sunderland*, (London: Whittaker, Treacher and Arnott, 1832), p.21.
35. Ibid.
36. Ibid, p.28.
37. Ibid, p.34.
38. Ibid, p.35.
39. *The Times*, 12 November 1831.
40. Ibid.
41. William Reid Clanny, *Hyperanthraxis; Or, the Cholera of Sunderland*, (London: Whittaker, Treacher and Arnott, 1832), p.41.
42. Ibid.
43. *Morning Post,* 22 November 1831.
44. *The Times*, 12 November 1831.
45. National Research and Development Centre for adult literacy and numeracy; www.nrdc.org.uk/content.asp?CategoryID=602&ArticleID=467 [2014].
46. *The Times*, 15 November 1831.
47. Ibid.
48. *The Times*, 16 November 1831.
49. Ibid.
50. *The Times*, 5 December 1831.
51. *The Times*, 16 November 1831.
52. *The Times*, 5 December 1831.
53. *The Times*, 18 November 1831.
54. *Sheffield Independent*, 3 December 1831.
55. *The Times*, 23 December 1831.
56. *The Times*, 30 December 1831.
57. *The Times*, 21 December 1831.
58. *The Times*, 6 December 1831.
59. Ibid.
60. *Manchester Guardian*, 31 December 1831; The Guardian Archive, www. theguardian.com/theguardian/2012/jan/02/archive-spread-of-the-cholera-1831, [2014].
61. Amanda J. Thomas, *The Lambeth Cholera Outbreak of 1848-1849: The Setting, Causes, Course and Aftermath of an Epidemic in London,* (Jefferson, North Carolina: McFarland & Co., 2009), p. 77; *Lambeth Parish and Vestry Committee Minutes* (Ref.: P3), *Lambeth District Sanitary Reports* (Ref: P3, 73–75, 1848–1878); Lambeth Archives.
62. *The Times*, 24 January 1832.

# NOTES

63. Amanda J. Thomas, *The Lambeth Cholera Outbreak of 1848-1849: The Setting, Causes, Course and Aftermath of an Epidemic in London,* (Jefferson, North Carolina: McFarland & Co., 2009), p. 51; *The Times,*11 September 1849.

64. *The Times*, 30 December 1831.

65. Ibid

66. *Manchester Guardian*, 31 December 1831; The Guardian Archive, www.theguardian.com/theguardian/2012/jan/02/archive-spread-of-the-cholera-1831 [2014].

67. *The Times*, 30 December 1831.

68. Michael Dunnill, *Dr William Budd, Bristol's most famous physician*, (Bristol: Redcliffe, 2006), pp.20-21.

69. R.W. Sturgess, The *Great Age of Industry in the North East*, (Durham County Local History Society, 1981).

70. John G. Avery, *The Cholera Years. An Account of the Cholera Outbreaks in our Ports, Towns and Villages* (Southampton: Beech Books, 2001).

71. S.T. Anning, 'Leeds House of Recovery,' (http://europepmc.org/articles/PMC1033950/pdf/medhist00138-0018.pdf□ 1969 [2014]).

72. *The Times*, 10 February 1832.

73. Andrew Miller; *The Rise And Progress Of Coatbridge And Surrounding Neighbourhood, Dundyvan Iron Works, Glasgow 1864,* www.scottishmining.co.uk/415.html [2014].

74. R.W. Sturgess, The *Great Age of Industry in the North East*, (Durham County Local History Society, 1981).

75. Anthony Burton, *Canal 250. The Story of Britain's Canals*, (Stroud, Glos.: The History Press, 2011).

76. *The Glass Industry of Tyne and Wear; Part One: Glassmaking on Wearside*, (Tyne and Wear County Council (Museums), 1979; L/PA/146).

77. *The Times*, 18 August 1832.

78. M. Durey, *The First Spasmodic Cholera Epidemic in York, 1832* (York: St Anthony's Press, 1974), p.5.

79. Ibid.

80. *York Herald*, 9 June, 1832; www.findmypast.co.uk

81. J. P. Needham, *Facts and observations relative to the disease commonly called cholera, as it has recently prevailed in the city of York*, (London: Longman, Rees, Orme, Brown, Green, and Co, 1833), p.107.

82. *York Herald*, 9 June, 1832; www.findmypast.co.uk

83. *Yorkshire Gazette*, 23 June 1832; www.findmypast.co.uk

84. York History, (www.yorkhistory.org.uk/node/78), [2014].

85. *Wolverhampton Chronicle*, 31 January 1849, from a lecture, 30 January 1849, by Rev. J. B. Owen, Vicar of Saint Marys, Bilston, www.wolverhamptonhistory.org.uk/politics/health/public/diseases [2014].

86. Marc Alexander, *The Sutton Companion to the Folklore, Myths and Customs of Britain*, (Stroud, Glos.: The History Press, 2005).

87. From a poster, dated 1848, 'Memorial of the Cholera which visited BILSTON, in the Year of Our Lord, 1832,' www.sharehistory.org/janes/uploads/5970-bilston-cholera-epidemic [2014].

88. Norman Longmate, *King Cholera. The Biography of a Disease,* (London: Hamish Hamilton, 1966, p.111.

89. R.W. Sturgess, *The Great Age of Industry in the North East*, (Durham County Local History Society, 1981).

90. *The Times,* 14 February 1832.

91. Michael Dunnill, *Dr William Budd, Bristol's most famous physician*, (Bristol: Redcliffe, 2006), p.80.

92. Thomas Shapter, *The History of the Cholera in Exeter in 1832*, (Wakefield and London: S.R. Publishers Ltd., 1971), p.78.

93. Ibid, pp.75-8.

94. Norman Longmate, *King Cholera. The Biography of a Disease,* (London: Hamish Hamilton, 1966), p.121.

95. Thomas Shapter, *The History of the Cholera in Exeter in 1832*, (Wakefield and London: S.R. Publishers Ltd., 1971), pp.241-235.

96. Michael Dunnill, *Dr William Budd, Bristol's most famous physician*, (Bristol: Redcliffe, 2006), p.79.

97. UK Parliament Website; www.parliament.uk/about/living-heritage/ trans formingsociety/towncountry/towns/tyne-and-wear-case-study/introduction/cholera-in-sunderland [2014].

98. Thomas Shapter, *The History of the Cholera in Exeter in 1832*, (Wakefield and London: S.R. Publishers Ltd., 1971), Robert Newton, 'Introduction,' p. v.

99. Thomas Snow, (1888), 'Doctor's teetotal address delivered in 1836.' (*The British Temperance Advocate,*), http://johnsnow.matrix.msu.edu/work.php?id=15-78-1 [2014].

100. *The Times*, 25 June 1849.

101. *The Times*, 26 June 1849.

102. *The Times*, 1 November 1848.

**Chapter 3 The Wretched State of the Poor**
1. Cathryn Tonne, Paul Wilkinson, (2013) 'Long-term exposure to air pollution is associated with survival following acute coronary syndrome,' *European Heart Journal*, http://eurheartj.oxfordjournals.org/content/early/2013/02/18/eurheartj.ehs480 [2014].

2. Clive Behagg, *Labour and Reform, Working-Class Movements 1815-1914*, (London: Hodder and Stoughton, 1991), p.1.

3. Chris Cook, *The Routledge Companion to Britain in the Nineteenth Century, 1815-1914*, (Routledge, 2005), p.103.

4. Michael Dunnill, *Dr William Budd, Bristol's most famous physician*, (Bristol: Redcliffe, 2006), p.13.

5. John Atkinson Hobson, *Problems of Poverty: An Inquiry Into the Industrial Condition of the Poor,* (RareBooksClub.com, 2012), p.2.

6. Gilbert Blaine, *A Warning to the British Public Against the Alarming Approach of the Indian cholera and the History of the Epidemic Cholera of India, from its first appearance in the year 1817, to 1831, and the dreadful ravages it has committed, with the dates of its first appearance in the different provinces,* (London: Burgess and Hill, 1831), pp.1-14.

7. Paul Theerman, 'Calculating Lifetimes: Life Expectancy and Medical Progress at the Turn of the Century,' August 2014; Books, Health and History, the New York Academy of Medicine; http://nyamcenterforhistory.org/tag/william-farr [2014].

8. Val Curtis et al., (2011), 'Hygiene: new hopes, new horizons,' The *Lancet, Infectious*

210

*Diseases*, 11(4), pp. 312-21, www.ncbi.nlm.nih.gov/pubmed/21453872 [2014].

9. V. Curtis, S. Cairncross, (2003), 'Effect of washing hand with soap on diarrhoea risk in the community: a systematic review,' The *Lancet, Infectious Diseases*, 3(5), pp. 275-81 (Abstract), www.ncbi.nlm.nih.gov/pubmed/12726975 [2014].

10. Chris Cook, *The Routledge Companion to Britain in the Nineteenth Century, 1815-1914*, (London: Routledge, 2005), p. 103.

11. Dr John Simon, *Report on the last two Cholera-Epidemics of London, as affected by the consumption of impure water,* (Eyre and Spottiswood, 1856).

12. Richard Rodger, *Housing in Urban Britain 1780-1914,* (Cambridge University Press, 1995), pp.32-4.

13. Ibid.

14. M.W. Flinn, *Introduction; Report on The Sanitary Condition of the Labouring Population of Great Britain by Edwin Chadwick, 1842;* (Edinburgh University Press, 1965), pp. 5-6.

15. Amanda J. Thomas, *The Lambeth Cholera Outbreak of 1848-1849: The Setting, Causes, Course and Aftermath of an Epidemic in London,* (Jefferson, North Carolina: McFarland & Co., 2009), p.136.

16. Michael Dunnill, *Dr William Budd, Bristol's most famous physician*, (Bristol: Redcliffe, 2006), pp.48-9.

17. David Gibbons, *The Metropolitan Buildings Act. 7th & 8th. Vict. Cap. 84. With Notes and an Index*, (London: Weale, 1844), pp.146-7.

18. Stephen Halliday, *The Great Stink of London. Sir Joseph Bazalgette and the Cleansing of the Victorian Metropolis* (Stroud, Glos.: Sutton, 2007), p.47.

19. Eric C. Midwinter, *Social Administration in Lancashire, 1830-1860: Poor Law, Public Health and Police*, (Manchester University Press, 1969), p.84.

20. G. N. Olsen, et al., (1998) 'Liverpool's drainage history: seventeenth century to MEPAS,' *Municipal Engineer*, 121, (2), 67-77; www.icevirtuallibrary.com/content/article/10.1680/imuen.1997.29487 [2014].

21. 'Housing and Health in Liverpool a History,' www.liverpoolpicturebook.com/2012/10/HousingandHealthLiverpool.html [2014].

22. Dr William Cunningham Glen, *The Nuisances Removal and Diseases Prevention Acts, 1848 & 1849*, (Third Edition, London: Shaw and Sons, 1849), p.4.

23. Metropolitan Commission of Sewers, *Administrative Papers, 1847-1862,* http://discovery.nationalarchives.gov.uk/details/rd/6cd47612-3a72-465c-a68b-eab8e927362f [2014].

24. William A. Robson, *The Government and Misgovernment of London*, (London: Routledge, 2013), p.122.

25. Christopher Hamlin, *Public Health and Social Justice in the Age of Chadwick: Britain, 1800-1854,* (Cambridge, New York, Melbourne: Cambridge University Press, 1998), p.310.

26. Amanda J. Thomas, *The Lambeth Cholera Outbreak of 1848-1849: The Setting, Causes, Course and Aftermath of an Epidemic in London,* (Jefferson, North Carolina: McFarland & Co., 2009), p. 65; Edwin Chadwick, David Gladstone, and Samuel Edward Finer, *Edwin Chadwick: Nineteenth-century Social Reform* (London: Routledge,1997), p. 335.

27. Stephen Halliday, *The Great Stink of London. Sir Joseph Bazalgette and the Cleansing of the Victorian Metropolis* (Stroud: Sutton, 2007), p.49.

28. Amanda J. Thomas, *The Lambeth Cholera Outbreak of 1848-1849: The Setting, Causes, Course and Aftermath of an Epidemic in London,* (Jefferson, North Carolina: McFarland & Co., 2009), p.64.

29. Stephen Halliday, *The Great Stink of London. Sir Joseph Bazalgette and the Cleansing of the Victorian Metropolis* (Stroud: Sutton, 2007), p.49.

30. Amanda J. Thomas, *The Lambeth Cholera Outbreak of 1848-1849: The Setting, Causes, Course and Aftermath of an Epidemic in London,* (Jefferson, North Carolina: McFarland & Co., 2009), p.201; Edwin Chadwick, David Gladstone, and Samuel Edward Finer, *Edwin Chadwick: Nineteenth-century Social Reform* (London: Routledge, 1997), p.364.

31. Stephen Halliday, *The Great Stink of London. Sir Joseph Bazalgette and the Cleansing of the Victorian Metropolis* (Stroud: Sutton, 2007), pp.51-2.

32. 'Obituary, Frank Forster, 1800-1852,' *Minutes of the Proceedings*, 12, (1853), p.153, www.icevirtuallibrary.com/content/article/10.1680/imotp.1853.23977 [2014].

33. Stephen Halliday, *The Great Stink of London. Sir Joseph Bazalgette and the Cleansing of the Victorian Metropolis* (Stroud: Sutton, 2007), p.55.

34. Ibid, pp.55-6.

35. S. G. and E. A. O. Checkland *The Poor Law Report of 1834*, (Penguin, 1974), p.19.

36. Ibid, p.67.

37. Ibid, pp.29-31.

38. Christopher Hamlin, 'Public Health Then and Now. Could You Starve to Death in England in 1839? The Chadwick-Farr Controversy and the Loss of the "Social" in Public Health,' (*American Journal of Public Health*, June 1995, Vol. 85, No. 6), p.857.

39. S.G. and E.A.O. Checkland *The Poor Law Report of 1834*, (Penguin Books, 1974), p.35.

40. Ibid, pp.122-3.

41. Ibid, p.335.

42. Ibid, p.375.

43. Ibid, pp.38-43; 478.

44. Amanda J. Thomas, *The Lambeth Cholera Outbreak of 1848-1849: The Setting, Causes, Course and Aftermath of an Epidemic in London,* (Jefferson, North Carolina: McFarland & Co., 2009), p.54; *Enlightenment Scotland* www.educationscotland.gov.uk/scottishenlightenment/scotland [2014].

45. Robert B. Ekelund, Edward O. Price, *The Economics of Edwin Chadwick: Incentives Matter*, (Cheltenham: Edward Elgar Publishing, 2012), p.10.

46. Chadwick, Sir Edwin (1800–1890), www.oxforddnb.com/index/101005013/Edwin-Chadwick [2014].

47. Ralph R. Frerichs, *Brief History During the Snow Era*, www.ph.ucla.edu/epi/snow/1859map/chadwick_edwin_a2.html [2014].

48. Chadwick, Sir Edwin (1800–1890), www.oxforddnb.com/index/101005013/Edwin-Chadwick [2014].

49. J. H. Burns, *Happiness and Utility: Jeremy Bentham's Equation*, (University College London www.utilitarianism.com/jeremy-bentham/greatest-happiness.pdf ), p.1;

50. *Online Guide to Ethics and Moral Philosophy; Utilitarian Theories* (1996), http://caae.phil.cmu.edu/Cavalier/80130/part2/sect9.html [2014].

51. Christopher Hamlin, 'Public Health Then and Now. Could You Starve to Death in England in 1839? The Chadwick-Farr Controversy and the Loss of the "Social" in

# NOTES

Public Health,' (*American Journal of Public Health*, June 1995, Vol. 85, No. 6), p.862.

52. *The 1833 Factory Act*, www.parliament.uk/about/living-heritage/transformingsociety/livinglearning/19thcentury/overview/factoryact [2014].

53. Amanda J. Thomas, *The Lambeth Cholera Outbreak of 1848-1849: The Setting, Causes, Course and Aftermath of an Epidemic in London*, (Jefferson, North Carolina: McFarland & Co., 2009), p.56.

54. Rosemary Rees, *Poverty and Public Health, 1815-1948*, (Oxford: Heinemann, 2001), p.134.

55. Ibid.

56. William Laxton, (1850), *The Civil Engineer and Architect's Journal*, 13, pp.139-40.

57. Rosemary Rees, *Poverty and Public Health, 1815-1948*, (Oxford: Heinemann, 2001), p.133.

58. M.W. Flinn, *Introduction; Report on The Sanitary Condition of the Labouring Population of Great Britain* by Edwin Chadwick, 1842; (Edinburgh University Press, 1965), p.210.

59. Ibid, pp.47–52.

60. Ibid, p.60.

61. Ibid, pp.67-8.

62. George Rosen, *A History of Public Health*, (Baltimore, Maryland, John Hopkins University Press, 1993), p.194.

63. (2012) *UCL Bloomsbury Project*, www.ucl.ac.uk/bloomsbury-project [2014].

64. George Rosen, *A History of Public Health*, (Baltimore, Maryland, John Hopkins University Press, 1993), p.194.

65. Ibid, p.196.

66. www.workhouses.org.uk

67. Rosemary Rees, *Poverty and Public Health, 1815-1948*, (Oxford: Heinemann, 2001), p.134.

68. George Rosen, *A History of Public Health*, (Baltimore, Maryland, John Hopkins University Press, 1993), p.196.

69. Amanda J. Thomas, *The Lambeth Cholera Outbreak of 1848-1849: The Setting, Causes, Course and Aftermath of an Epidemic in London*, (Jefferson, North Carolina: McFarland & Co., 2009), p.66.

70. George Rosen, *A History of Public Health*, (Baltimore, Maryland, John Hopkins University Press, 1993), p.197.

71. Chadwick, Sir Edwin (1800–1890), www.oxforddnb.com/index/101005013/Edwin-Chadwick [2014].

72. Amanda J. Thomas, *The Lambeth Cholera Outbreak of 1848-1849: The Setting, Causes, Course and Aftermath of an Epidemic in London*, (Jefferson, North Carolina: McFarland & Co., 2009), p.66.

73. George Rosen, *A History of Public Health*, (Baltimore, Maryland, John Hopkins University Press, 1993), p.197.

74. Ibid, p.198.

75. Mike Billington, *Using the Building Regulations: Administrative Procedures*, (Routledge, 2006), p.16.

76. The Oxford Dictionary of National Biography; www.oxforddnb.com

77. *Report from His Majesty's Commissioners for Inquiring into the Administration and Practical Operation of the Poor Laws*, (London: HM Stationery Office, 1834), p.181.

**Chapter 4 Cholera and Tooting's Pauper Paradise**

1. Peter Higginbotham, (2014), *Mr Drouet's Establishment for Pauper Children, Tooting,* www.workhouses.org.uk/Drouet [2014]; (2010), *London Lives 1690 to 1800 - Crime, Poverty and Social Policy in the Metropolis,* www.londonlives.org/static/ParliamentaryReform.jsp [2014].

2. Merton Historical Society.

3. *The Times*, 20 January 1849.

4. *The Times*, 19 January 1849.

5. (2013), *The Proceedings of the Old Bailey, London's Central Criminal Court, 1674 to 1913,* www.oldbaileyonline.org/browse.jsp?id=def1-919-18490409&div=t18490409-919&terms=tooting#highlight [2014].

6. *The Times*, 8 January 1849.

7. B. R. Curle, *Mr Drouet's Establishment at Tooting: an Essay in Victorian Child Welfare,* http://archaeologydataservice.ac.uk/archiveDS [2014].

8. *The Times*, 20 January 1849.

9. *1841 Census*, 1068, 6, p.1, (Accessed via Ancestry, www.ancestry.co.uk) [2014].

10. *The Times*, 20 January 1849.

11. *The Times*, 13, 19, 20 January 1849.

12. *The Times*, 26 January 1849.

13. B. R. Curle, *Mr Drouet's Establishment at Tooting: an Essay in Victorian Child Welfare,* http://archaeologydataservice.ac.uk/archiveDS [2014].

14. *1841 Census*, 1068, 6, p.1, (Accessed via Ancestry, www.ancestry.co.uk) [2014].

15. *The Times*, 17 January 1849.

16. *The Times*, 26 January 1849.

17. General Register Office, England.

18. (2013), *The Proceedings of the Old Bailey, London's Central Criminal Court, 1674 to 1913,* www.oldbaileyonline.org/browse.jsp?id=def1-919-18490409&div=t18490409-919&terms=tooting#highlight [2014].

19. *The Times*, 20 January, 1849.

20. Ibid.

21. *The Times*, 13 January, 1849.

22. The Times, 24 January 1849.

23. *The Times*, 13 January, 1849.

24. *The Times*, 20 January, 1849.

25. *The Times*, 4 January 1849.

26. R. J. Morris, (1977), 'Cholera 1832 – The Social Response to An Epidemic,' *Medical History*, 21(3), p.336, www.ph.ucla.edu/epi/snow/morris/morris_lessons_a.html [2014].

27. *The Times*, 13 January 1849.

28. Erwin H. Ackerknecht, 'Anticontagionism Between 1821 and 1867,' The Fielding H. Garrison Lecture, (*International Journal of Epidemiology*, Vol. 38, Issue 1), pp. 7-21.

29. *The Times*, 8 January 1849.

30. *The Times*, 16 January 1849.

31. *The Times*, 13 January 1849.

32. Ibid.

33. *The Times*, 8 January 1849.

34. *The Times*, 13 January 1849.

35. *The Times*, 8, and 19 January 1849.
36. (2013), *The Proceedings of the Old Bailey, London's Central Criminal Court, 1674 to 1913*, www.oldbaileyonline.org/browse.jsp?id=def1-919-18490409&div=t18490409-919&terms=tooting#highlight [2014].
37. *The Times*, 19 and 20 January 1849.
38. *The Times*, 19 January 1849.
39. (2013), *The Proceedings of the Old Bailey, London's Central Criminal Court, 1674 to 1913*, www.oldbaileyonline.org/browse.jsp?id=def1-919-18490409&div=t18490409-919&terms=tooting#highlight [2014].
40. *The Times*, 20 January 1849.
41. *The Times*, 17 January 1849.
42. *The Times*, 20 January 1849.
43. *The Times*, 13 January 1849.
44. *The Times*, 20 January 1849.
45. *The Times*, 17 and 20 January 1849.
46. *The Times*, 20 January 1849.
47. (2013), *The Proceedings of the Old Bailey, London's Central Criminal Court, 1674 to 1913*, www.oldbaileyonline.org/browse.jsp?id=def1-919-18490409&div=t18490409-919&terms=tooting#highlight [2014].
48. Druin Burch, *Digging up the Dead, Uncovering the Life and Times of an Extraordinary Surgeon,* (London: Vintage, 2007).
49. *The Times,* 11 January 1849.
50. *The Times*, 19 January 1849.
51. Ibid.
52. *The Times*, 20 January 1849.
53. Peter Higginbotham, (2014), *Mr Drouet's Establishment for Pauper Children, Tooting,* www.workhouses.org.uk/Drouet [2014].
54. *The Times*, 24 January 1849.
55. Ibid.
56. Ibid.
57. Ibid.
58. *The Times*, 1 February 1849.
59. (2013), *The Proceedings of the Old Bailey, London's Central Criminal Court, 1674 to 1913*, www.oldbaileyonline.org/browse.jsp?id=def1-919-18490409&div=t18490409-919&terms=tooting#highlight [2014].
60. Ibid.
61. *The Examiner,* 23 April 1849, (The Workhouse, www.workhouses.org.uk).
62. *Dundee Courier*, 1 August 1849.
63. Ibid.
64. Charles Dickens, (1849), 'The Paradise at Tooting,' *The Examiner,* www.workhouses.org.uk/Drouet/Examiner1.shtml [2014].
65. (Accessed via Ancestry, www.ancestry.co.uk) [2014].
66. *Evening Standard*, 19 February 1849.
67. (Accessed via Ancestry, www.ancestry.co.uk) [2014].
68. 'Report from His Majesty's Commissioners for Inquiring into the Administration and Practical Operation of the Poor Laws, 1834,' (*London Gazette*, 1834), p.192.
69. Andrew Roberts, (1991), *England's Poor Law Commissioners and the Trade in*

*Pauper Lunacy, 1834-1847,* http://studymore.org.uk/mott.htm [2014].
70. Friedrich Engels, *The Condition of the Working Class in England,* (London: Penguin Classics, 2005), p.223.
71. *1841 Census,* 1050, 9, 27, p.1, (Accessed via Ancestry, www.ancestry.co.uk) [2014].
72.Peter Higginbotham, (2014), *The Lancet Reports on Metropolitan Workhouse Infirmaries, 1865-66: Camberwell,* www.workhouses.org.uk/Lancet/Camberwell.shtml [2014].

**Chapter 5 Births, Marriages and Deaths**
1. Chris Cook, *The Routledge Companion to Britain in the Nineteenth Century, 1815-1914,* (London: Routledge, 2005), p.103.
2. Ibid, p.104.
3. Julie Jefferies, *Focus On, People and Migration The UK population: past, present and future,* (Office for National Statistics, 2005), pp.1-4.
4. T. R. Malthus, *An Essay on the Principle of Population,* (Oxford University Press, 2008), p.61.
5. Colin G. Pooley, and Jean Turnbull, *Migration and Mobility in Britain Since the 18th Century,* (London: Routledge, 1998), p. 279.
6. Margaret Pelling, *Cholera, Fever and English Medicine, 1825-1865,* (Oxford University Press, 1978), p.82; Bentham, *Works,* ix. 443-7.
7. Amanda J. Thomas, *The Lambeth Cholera Outbreak of 1848-1849: The Setting, Causes, Course and Aftermath of an Epidemic in London,* (Jefferson, North Carolina: McFarland & Co., 2009), p.25.
8. Duncan Watts, *Whigs, Radicals and Liberals 1815-1914,* (London: Hodder Murray, 2002), p.19.
9. *Who Was Jeremy Bentham?,* www.ucl.ac.uk/Bentham-Project/who [2014].
10. Daniel J. Friedman, Edward L. Hunter, R. Gibson Parrish, *Health Statistics: Shaping Policy and Practice to Improve the Population's Health,* (Oxford University Press, 2005), p.30.
11. Ibid.
12. Margaret Pelling, *Cholera, Fever and English Medicine, 1825-1865,* (Oxford University Press, 1978), p.98.
13. Civil Registration, www.1837.com/civil-registration [2014].
14. (Accessed via Findmypast, www.findmypast.co.uk) [2014].
15. Civil Registration, www.1837.com/civil-registration [2014].
16. Births and Deaths Registration Act 1874, www.legislation.gov.uk/ukpga/Vict/37-38/88/contents [2014].
17. John M. Eyler, (1973), 'William Farr on the Cholera: The Sanitarian's Disease Theory and the Statistician's Method,' *Journal of the History of Medicine,* p.80, www.medicine.mcgill.ca/epidemiology/hanley/temp/material/SnowCholera/EyleronWilliamFarrCholera.pdf [2014].
18. Dorothy Porter, *Health, Civilization and the State: A History of Public Health from Ancient to Modern Times,* (London: Routledge, 1999), p.70.
19. Margaret Pelling, *Cholera, Fever and English Medicine, 1825-1865,* (Oxford University Press, 1978), p.85.
20. John M. Eyler, (1973), 'William Farr on the Cholera: The Sanitarian's Disease Theory and the Statistician's Method,' *Journal of the History of Medicine,* p.80,

# NOTES

www.medicine.mcgill.ca/epidemiology/hanley/temp/material/SnowCholera/EyleronWilliamFarrCholera.pdf [2014].

21. P.M. Dunn, 'Perinatal lessons from the past; Dr William Farr of Shropshire (1807–1883): obstetric mortality and training,' (*Arch Dis Child Fetal Neonatal Ed* 2002; 87: F67-F69 doi:10.1136/fn.87.1.F67, 2002).

22. John M. Eyler, (1973), 'William Farr on the Cholera: The Sanitarian's Disease Theory and the Statistician's Method,' *Journal of the History of Medicine,* p.80, www.medicine.mcgill.ca/epidemiology/hanley/temp/material/SnowCholera/EyleronWilliamFarrCholera.pdf [2014].

23. Ibid, p.81.

24. M. Whitehead (2000), 'William Farr's Legacy to the Study of Inadequacies in Health,' *Bulletin of the World Health Organisation,* 78(1), p.1, www.ncbi.nlm.nih.gov/pmc/articles/PMC2560600/ [2014]; *Cholera, Fever and English Medicine, 1825-1865*, Margaret Pelling, Oxford University Press, 1978, p.83.

25. Daniel J. Friedman, Edward L. Hunter, R. Gibson Parrish, *Health Statistics: Shaping Policy and Practice to Improve the Population's Health,* (Oxford University Press, 2005), p.31.

26. Margaret Pelling, *Cholera, Fever and English Medicine, 1825-1865*, (Oxford University Press, 1978), p.82.

27. Thomas Shapter, *The History of the Cholera in Exeter in 1832*, (Wakefield and London: S.R. Publishers Ltd., 1971), p.175.

28. Daniel J. Friedman, Edward L. Hunter, R. Gibson Parrish, *Health Statistics: Shaping Policy and Practice to Improve the Population's Health,* (Oxford University Press, 2005), p.31.

29. Margaret Pelling, *Cholera, Fever and English Medicine, 1825-1865*, (Oxford University Press, 1978), p.98.

30. Ibid.

31. *London Standard*, 12 September 1849.

32. Ibid.

33. Christopher Hamlin, 'Public Health Then and Now. Could You Starve to Death in England in 1839? The Chadwick-Farr Controversy and the Loss of the "Social" in Public Health,' (*American Journal of Public Health*, June 1995, Vol. 85, No. 6), p.858.

34. Daniel J. Friedman, Edward L. Hunter, R. Gibson Parrish, *Health Statistics: Shaping Policy and Practice to Improve the Population's Health,* (Oxford University Press, 2005), p.31.

35. Margaret Pelling, *Cholera, Fever and English Medicine, 1825-1865*, (Oxford University Press, 1978), p.96.

36. Christopher Hamlin, 'Public Health Then and Now. Could You Starve to Death in England in 1839? The Chadwick-Farr Controversy and the Loss of the "Social" in Public Health,' (*American Journal of Public Health*, June 1995, Vol. 85, No. 6), p.859.

37. *Sir John Simon's Medical Officer of Health reports on the* Sanitary Condition of London, *1848-55*, Medical Officer of Health Reports 1848-9, pp.6-7, http://ewds.strath.ac.uk/historymedicine/View/Resource/tabid/6225/articleType/ArticleView/articleId/781/Sir-John-Simons-Medical-Officer-of-Health-reports-on-the-Sanitary-Condition-of-London-1848-55.aspx [2014].

38. Daniel J. Friedman, Edward L. Hunter, R. Gibson Parrish, *Health Statistics:*

*Shaping Policy and Practice to Improve the Population's Health,* (Oxford University Press, 2005), p.31.

39. Raymond Flood, Adrian Rice, Robin Wilson, *Mathematics in Victorian Britain*, (Oxford University Press, 2011), p.281.

40. John M. Eyler, (1973), 'William Farr on the Cholera: The Sanitarian's Disease Theory and the Statistician's Method,' *Journal of the History of Medicine,* p.97, www.medicine.mcgill.ca/epidemiology/hanley/temp/material/SnowCholera/EyleronWil liamFarrCholera.pdf [2014].

41. Daniel J. Friedman, Edward L. Hunter, R. Gibson Parrish, *Health Statistics: Shaping Policy and Practice to Improve the Population's Health,* (Oxford University Press, 2005), p.31.

42. Margaret Pelling, *Cholera, Fever and English Medicine, 1825-1865,* (Oxford University Press, 1978), p.91.

43. William Farr, *Report on the Mortality of Cholera in England 1848-9,* (London: W. Clowes and Sons, 1852), p.lxix, http://pds.lib.harvard.edu/pds/view/8278007?n=9&imagesize=1200&jp2Res=.25&print Thumbnails=no [2014]

44. Ibid.

45. William Farr, *Report on the Mortality of Cholera in England 1848-9,* (London: W. Clowes and Sons, 1852), p.lxxii, http://pds.lib.harvard.edu/pds/view/8278007?n=9&imagesize=1200&jp2Res=.25&print Thumbnails=no [2014].

46. Ibid, p.v.

47. John M. Eyler, (1973), 'William Farr on the Cholera: The Sanitarian's Disease Theory and the Statistician's Method,' *Journal of the History of Medicine,* pp.79-80, www.medicine.mcgill.ca/epidemiology/hanley/temp/material/SnowCholera/EyleronWil liamFarrCholera.pdf [2014].

48. Ibid, p.83.

**Chapter 6 The Graveyards Overflow**
1. *Rosary Cemetery Chapel, Norwich,* www.norfolkchurches.co.uk/norwichrosary/norwichrosary.htm [2014].

2.*Westgate Hill Cemetery,* http://list.english-heritage.org.uk/resultsingle.aspx?uid=1001680 [2014].

3. John G. Avery, *The Cholera Years. An Account of the Cholera Outbreaks in our Ports, Towns and Villages* (Southampton: Beech Books, 2001), p.79.

4. *London Standard,* 13 July 1831.

5. Amanda J. Thomas, *The Lambeth Cholera Outbreak of 1848-1849: The Setting, Causes, Course and Aftermath of an Epidemic in London,* (Jefferson, North Carolina: McFarland & Co., 2009), p.173.

6. Catharine Arnold, *Necropolis: London and Its Dead,* (London: Simon & Schuster, 2006), p.125.

7. *Paul, Sir John Dean, second baronet (1802–1868), banker and fraudster* www.oxforddnb.com/index/101021602/John-Dean-Paul [2014].

8. *London Standard,* 13 July 1831.

9. Catharine Arnold, *Necropolis: London and Its Dead,* (London: Simon & Schuster, 2006), pp.125-6.

10. *London Standard*, 13 July 1831.

11. Catharine Arnold, *Necropolis: London and Its Dead*, (London: Simon & Schuster, 2006), pp.126; London Metropolitan Archives, ref. GB 0074 b/GC.

12. *Church Cemetery*, http://list.english-heritage.org.uk/resultsingle.aspx?uid=1001486

13. *London Gazette*, 15 November 1831, issue 18876, p.2424.

14. *London Medical Gazette: or, Journal of Practical Medicine*, Volume 9, (London: Longman, 1832), p. 406.

15. *Sussex Advertiser*, 19 December 1931.

16. Simon C. Wilkinson, *Cholera Deaths, Burials in July & August 1832*, www.upton.uk.net/history/genealogy/cholera.html [2014].

17. (2007), *English Heritage, PastScape*; (Accessed via http://pastscape.org) [2014].

18. Simon C. Wilkinson, *Cholera Deaths, Burials in July & August 1832*, www.upton.uk.net/history/genealogy/cholera.html [2014].

19. *Monument Grounds, Sheffield*, http://list.english-heritage.org.uk/resultsingle.aspx?uid=1000284 [2014].

20. Norman Longmate, *King Cholera. The Biography of a Disease* (London: Hamish Hamilton, 1966), p.89.

21. M. Durey, *The First Spasmodic Cholera Epidemic in York, 1832* (York: St Anthony's Press, 1974), p.7.

22. Norman Longmate, *King Cholera. The Biography of a Disease* (London: Hamish Hamilton, 1966), pp.121-2.

23. Thomas Shapter, *The History of the Cholera in Exeter in 1832*, (Wakefield and London: S.R. Publishers Ltd., 1971), p.173.

24. Ibid, pp.235-7.

25. Ibid, p.173.

26. Ibid, p.175.

27. Ibid, p.145.

28. Ibid, p.169.

29. *Gloucester Citizen*, 8 July 1884.

30. George Alfred Walker, *Gatherings from Grave Yards, Particularly Those of London: with a Concise History of the Modes of Interment Among Different Nations, from the Earliest Periods. And a Detail of Dangerous and Fatal Results Produced by the Unwise and Revolting Custom of Inhuming the Dead in the Midst of the Living*, (London: Longman and Co., 1839), pp.167-9.

31. Ibid, pp.154-6.

32. (1877), 'Burial Acts Consolidation Bill,' Hansard, http://hansard.millbanksystems.com/lords/1877/mar/13/bill-presented-first-reading [2014].

33. Catharine Arnold, *Necropolis: London and Its Dead*, (London: Simon & Schuster, 2006), p.115.

34. Edwin Chadwick, *Report on the Sanitary Condition of the Labouring Population of Great Britain. A Supplementary Re[port On the Results of a Special Inquiry into the Practice of Interment in Towns*, (London: W. Clowes, 1843), pp.197-201.

35. Sylvia M. Barnard, *To Prove I'm Not Forgot: Living and Dying in a Victorian City*, (Manchester University Press, 1990), p.197.

36. *The Times*, 26 October 1849.

37. *London Daily News*, 15 November 1849.

38. Pam Fisher, 'Houses for the Dead: The Provision of Mortuaries in London, 1843–

1889,' (*The London Journal*, Vol. 34 No. 1, March, 2009,) pp.1–15.
39. *The Burial Board Acts of England and Wales*, (London: William Cunningham Glen, Shaw and Sons, 1868,), 16 & 17 Vict. Cap. 134, pp.80-1; https://archive.org/stream/burial boardacts00glengoog/burialboardacts00glengoog_djvu.txt [2014].
40. *The Times*, 19 January 1854.
41. Lambeth Landmark (Lambeth Archives image collection), http://landmark.lambeth.gov.uk [2014].

**Chapter 7 Dr John Snow and the Removal of the Pump Handle**
1. Peter Vinten-Johansen, et al., *Cholera, Chloroform, and the Science of Medicine: A Life of John Snow*, (Oxford University Press USA, 2003), p.395.
2. Sedgwick, W. T. (William Thompson), *Principles of sanitary science and the public health with special reference to the causation and prevention of infectious diseases*, (New York: The Macmillan Company, 1902), p.170.
3. Tom Koch, *John Snow, Hero of Cholera, RIP*, (*Snow's Legacy: Epidemiology Today and Tomorrow*, The London School of Hygiene & Tropical Medicine, 16 March 2013).
4. Tom Koch, Kenneth Denike, (2009), 'Crediting his critics' concerns: Remaking John Snow's map of Broad Street cholera, 1854,' *Social Science & Medicine*, 69(8) pp.1246–1251, www.elsevier.com [2014].
5. Tom Koch, *John Snow, Hero of Cholera, RIP*, (*Snow's Legacy: Epidemiology Today and Tomorrow*, The London School of Hygiene & Tropical Medicine, 16 March 2013).
6. Ibid.
7. Peter Vinten-Johansen, et al., *Cholera, Chloroform, and the Science of Medicine: A Life of John Snow*, (Oxford University Press USA, 2003), pp.14-22.
8. Ibid, p.45.
9. David Zuck, *Charles Empson*, p.14, http://kora.matrix.msu.edu/files/21/120/15-78-18B-22-Empsonbiogdefin05.pdf, [2014].
10. Ralph R. Frerichs, *The Mysterious Uncle*, www.ph.ucla.edu/epi/snow/empson.html [2014].
11. Peter Vinten-Johansen, et al., *Cholera, Chloroform, and the Science of Medicine: A Life of John Snow*, (Oxford University Press USA, 2003), p.30.
12. Royal College of Surgeons, (2012), *Plarr's Lives of the Fellows Online*, Greenhow, Thomas Michael, http://livesonline.rcseng.ac.uk/biogs/E002048b.htm [2014].
13. Peter Vinten-Johansen, et al., *Cholera, Chloroform, and the Science of Medicine: A Life of John Snow*, (Oxford University Press USA, 2003), p.42.
14. John Snow, *On the Mode of Communication of Cholera*, (London: John Churchill, 1855), p.20.
15. Peter Vinten-Johansen, et al., *Cholera, Chloroform, and the Science of Medicine: A Life of John Snow*, (Oxford University Press USA, 2003), p.44.
16. John Frank Newton, *The Return to Nature: or, A defence of the vegetable regimen; with some account of an experiment made during the last three or four years in the author's family, Volume 6*, (London: T. Cadell and W. Davies, 1811); pp.iii-iv.
17. Peter Vinten-Johansen, et al., *Cholera, Chloroform, and the Science of Medicine: A Life of John Snow*, (Oxford University Press USA, 2003), p.47.
18. Thomas Snow, (1888), 'Doctor's teetotal address delivered in 1836.' (*The British Temperance Advocate*,), http://johnsnow.matrix.msu.edu/work.php?id=15-78-1 [2014].
19. Amanda J. Thomas, *The Lambeth Cholera Outbreak of 1848-1849: The Setting,*

# NOTES

*Causes, Course and Aftermath of an Epidemic in London,* (Jefferson, North Carolina: McFarland & Co., 2009), p.207.

20. Stephanie J. Snow, (2000), 'John Snow MD (1813-1858). Part II: Becoming a doctor - his medical training and early years of practice,' *Journal of Medical Biography*, 8, pp.71-77, www.ph.ucla.edu/epi/snow/jmedbiography8_71_77_2000.pdf [2014].

21. Peter Vinten-Johansen, et al., *Cholera, Chloroform, and the Science of Medicine: A Life of John Snow*, (Oxford University Press USA, 2003), p.75.

22. Stephanie J. Snow, (2000), 'John Snow MD (1813-1858). Part II: Becoming a doctor - his medical training and early years of practice,' *Journal of Medical Biography*, 8, pp.71-77, www.ph.ucla.edu/epi/snow/jmedbiography8_71_77_2000.pdf [2014].

23. Peter Vinten-Johansen, et al., *Cholera, Chloroform, and the Science of Medicine: A Life of John Snow*, (Oxford University Press USA, 2003), pp. 81-84, pp.237-252.

24. Ibid, p.95.

25. Ibid, p.200.

26. Ibid, p.200-213.

27. Ralph R. Frerichs, 'Writings of John Snow at 36 Years of Age,' www.ph.ucla.edu/epi/snow/onpathmodecholera.html [2014].

28. Peter Vinten-Johansen, et al., *Cholera, Chloroform, and the Science of Medicine: A Life of John Snow*, (Oxford University Press USA, 2003), p.238.

29. Ibid, pp.246-251.

30. Ibid, p.257, p.395.

31. Tom Koch, *John Snow, Hero of Cholera, RIP*, (*Snow's Legacy: Epidemiology Today and Tomorrow*, The London School of Hygiene & Tropical Medicine, 16 March 2013).

32. John M. Eyler, (1973), 'William Farr on the Cholera: The Sanitarian's Disease Theory and the Statistician's Method,' *Journal of the History of Medicine*, p.91, www.medicine.mcgill.ca/epidemiology/hanley/temp/material/SnowCholera/EyleronWilliamFarrCholera.pdf [2014].

33. Stephen Halliday, *The War against Disease in Victorian England. The Great Filth*, (Stroud: Sutton, 2007), p.187.

34. John Snow, *On the Mode of Communication of Cholera*, (London: John Churchill, 1855), pp.59-60.

35. Ibid, pp.37-8.

36. (1855), *Report on the Cholera Outbreak in the Parish of St James, Westminster, during the Autumn of 1854*, The John Snow Archive and Research Companion, http://johnsnow.matrix.msu.edu/work.php?id=15-78-AA, [2014].

37. Ibid.

38. Ralph R. Frerichs, *Cholera in the Baltic Fleet*, www.ph.ucla.edu/epi/snow/cholerabalticfleet.html [2014].

39. *General Board of Health Report of the Committee for Scientific Inquiries in Relation to the Cholera-Epidemic of 1854*, (London: Eyre & Spottiswoode, 1855; The John Snow Archive and Research Companion; http://johnsnow.matrix.msu.edu/work.php?id=15-78-BE), pp.7-11.

40. John Snow, (1854), 'The Cholera near Golden-square, and Deptford,' *Medical Times and Gazette*, pp.321-22, http://johnsnow.matrix.msu.edu/work.php?id=15-78-45 [2014].

41. John Snow, *On the Mode of Communication of Cholera*, (London: John Churchill, 1855), p.40.

42. Ibid, pp.41-2.
43. Ibid, p.42.
44. Ibid, p.44.
45. Ibid.
46. Ibid.
47. Ibid, pp.41-2.
48. John Snow, (1854), 'The Cholera near Golden-square, and Deptford,' *Medical Times and Gazette,* pp.321-22, http://johnsnow.matrix.msu.edu/work.php?id=15-78-45 [2014].
49. John Snow, *On the Mode of Communication of Cholera,* (London: John Churchill, 1855), p.39.
50. John Snow, (1854), 'The Cholera near Golden-square, and Deptford,' *Medical Times and Gazette,* pp.321-22, http://johnsnow.matrix.msu.edu/work.php?id=15-78-45 [2014].
51. Peter Vinten-Johansen, et al., *Cholera, Chloroform, and the Science of Medicine: A Life of John Snow,* (Oxford University Press USA, 2003), pp.301-315.
52. Tom Koch, *Disease Maps, Epidemics on the Ground,* (University of Chicago Press, 2011).
53. Tom Koch, *Nobody loves a critic: Edmund A. Parkes and John Snow's cholera,* (Oxford University Press *International Journal of Epidemiology* 2013; 42: pp.1553–1559 doi:10.1093/ije/dyt194 _ The Author 2013).
54. Peter Vinten-Johansen, et al., *Cholera, Chloroform, and the Science of Medicine: A Life of John Snow,* (Oxford University Press USA, 2003), p.304.
55. (1854), *Report on the Cholera Outbreak in the Parish of St James, Westminster, during the Autumn of 1854,* http://johnsnow.matrix.msu.edu/work.php?id=15-78-AA [2014].
56. Peter Vinten-Johansen, et al., *Cholera, Chloroform, and the Science of Medicine: A Life of John Snow,* (Oxford University Press USA, 2003), p.310.
57. Charles Dickens, Jr., (1879), *Dickens's Dictionary of London,* www.victorianlondon.org/publications/dictionary.htm [2014].
58. (1854), *Report on the Cholera Outbreak in the Parish of St James, Westminster, during the Autumn of 1854,* http://johnsnow.matrix.msu.edu/work.php?id=15-78-AA [2014].
59. General Register Office, England.
60. (1854), *Report on the Cholera Outbreak in the Parish of St James, Westminster, during the Autumn of 1854,* http://johnsnow.matrix.msu.edu/work.php?id=15-78-AA [2014].
61. John Snow, (1854), 'The Cholera near Golden-square, and Deptford,' *Medical Times and Gazette,* pp.321-22, http://johnsnow.matrix.msu.edu/work.php?id=15-78-45 [2014].
62. (1854), *Report on the Cholera Outbreak in the Parish of St James, Westminster, during the Autumn of 1854,* http://johnsnow.matrix.msu.edu/work.php?id=15-78-AA [2014].
63. Ibid.
64. Ibid.
65. Edmund Cooper, *Report to the Metropolitan Commission of Sewers on the house-drainage in St. James, Westminster during the recent cholera outbreak,* 22 Sep 1854, (London Metropolitan Archives), pp.1-2.
66. Edwin Lankester, *Cholera: what is it? And How to Prevent it* (1866;

RareBooksClub.com, 2012), p.6.

67. E.A. Parkes, (1855), 'Review of Snow's Mode of Communication of Cholera,' British and Foreign Medical Review, pp. 449-63.
http://johnsnow.matrix.msu.edu/work.php?id=15-78-C1 [2014]

68. Ibid, p.458.

69. Ibid.

70. Tom Koch, *Nobody loves a critic: Edmund A. Parkes and John Snow's cholera,* (Oxford University Press
*International Journal of Epidemiology* 2013; 42: pp.1553–1559 doi:10.1093/ije/dyt194
_ The Author 2013.

71. E.A. Parkes, (1855), 'Review of Snow's Mode of Communication of Cholera,' British and Foreign Medical Review, pp. 449-63,
http://johnsnow.matrix.msu.edu/work.php?id=15-78-C1 [2014].

72. Metropolitan Sewage Committee Proceedings; *Parliamentary Papers*, 1846, 10, p.651, www.victorianlondon.org/disease/miasma.htm [2014].

73. Michael Dunnill, *Dr William Budd, Bristol's most famous physician*, (Bristol: Redcliffe, 2006), pp.14-15.

74. William Budd, 'Malignant Cholera: its cause, mode of propagation, and prevention,' *International Journal of Epidemiology* 2013;42:1567–1575, doi:10.1093/ije/dyt204, pp.1567-1574, http://ije.oxfordjournals.org/content/42/6/1567.short [2014].

75. Michael Dunnill, *Dr William Budd, Bristol's most famous physician*, (Bristol: Redcliffe, 2006), p.17.

76. Ibid, p.20.

77. Peter Vinten-Johansen, et al., *Cholera, Chloroform, and the Science of Medicine: A Life of John Snow*, (Oxford University Press USA, 2003), p.74.

78. William Budd, 'Malignant Cholera: its cause, mode of propagation, and prevention,' *International Journal of Epidemiology* 2013;42:1567–1575, doi:10.1093/ije/dyt204, p.1569, http://ije.oxfordjournals.org/content/42/6/1567.short [2014].

79. Michael Dunnill, *Dr William Budd, Bristol's most famous physician*, (Bristol: Redcliffe, 2006), pp.82-3.

80. William Budd, 'Malignant Cholera: its cause, mode of propagation, and prevention,' *International Journal of Epidemiology* 2013;42:1567–1575, doi:10.1093/ije/dyt204, p.1567, http://ije.oxfordjournals.org/content/42/6/1567.short [2014].

81. Ibid, p.1567.

82. Ibid.

83. Ibid.

84. Ibid.

85. Ibid, p.1568.

86. Ibid, p.1563.

87. Ibid, pp.1571-2.

88. Ibid, p.1572.

89. Margaret Pelling, *Cholera, Fever and English Medicine, 1825-1865*, (Oxford University Press, 1978), pp.151-162.

90. John Snow, *On the Mode of Communication of Cholera*, (London: John Churchill, 1855), p.52.

91. Margaret Pelling, *Cholera, Fever and English Medicine, 1825-1865*, (Oxford University Press, 1978), pp.156-158.

92. John M. Eyler, (1973), 'William Farr on the Cholera: The Sanitarian's Disease Theory and the Statistician's Method,' *Journal of the History of Medicine,* p.94, www.medicine.mcgill.ca/epidemiology/hanley/temp/material/SnowCholera/EyleronWil liamFarrCholera.pdf [2014].

93. (1855), *General Board of Health Report of the Committee for Scientific Inquiries in Relation to the Cholera-Epidemic of 1854,* p.52.
http://johnsnow.matrix.msu.edu/work.php?id=15-78-BE) [2014].

94. John Simon, (1856), *Report on the Last Two Cholera-Epidemics of London, as Affected by the Consumption of Impure Water,* pp.6-7.
http://johnsnow.matrix.msu.edu/work.php?id=15-78-7F [2014].

95. Walter Besant, *London in the Nineteenth Century*, (London: Forgotten Books, 2013; originally published 1909), p.357.

96. John Simon, (1856), *Report on the Last Two Cholera-Epidemics of London, as Affected by the Consumption of Impure Water,* pp.12-15,
http://johnsnow.matrix.msu.edu/work.php?id=15-78-7F [2014].

97. *The Times*, 26 June 1856.


**Chapter 8 The Stink of Cholera**

1. *The Times*, 5 June 1858.

2. William Baly and William Withey Gull, *Report on the Nature and Import of Certain Microscopic Bodies Found in the Intestinal Discharges of Cholera: Presented to the Cholera Committee of the Royal College of Physicians...by Their Sub-committee, on the 17th October, 1849*, Cholera Committee, Royal College of Physicians (London: John Churchill,1849), pp.20–21.

3. *The Times*, 15 June 1858.

4. *The Times*, 12 June 1858.

5. *The Times*, 2 July 1858.

6. Stephen Halliday, *The Great Stink of London. Sir Joseph Bazalgette and the Cleansing of the Victorian Metropolis* (Stroud: Sutton, 2007), p.63.

7. Stephen Halliday, *The War against Disease in Victorian England. The Great Filth,* (Stroud: Sutton, 2007), p. 205.

8. *The Times*, 21 June 1858.

9. Stephen Halliday, *The Great Stink of London. Sir Joseph Bazalgette and the Cleansing of the Victorian Metropolis* (Stroud, Glos.: Sutton, 2007), p.73.

10. *London Underground 150: Metropolitan line,*
www.ice.org.uk/topics/transport/London-Underground-150/Metropolitan-line [2015].

11. Stephen Halliday, *The Great Stink of London. Sir Joseph Bazalgette and the Cleansing of the Victorian Metropolis* (Stroud, Glos.: Sutton, 2007), pp.82-3; The Metropolitan Board of Works, *Annual Report* (1856-7), p.7.

12. Stephen Halliday, *The Great Stink of London. Sir Joseph Bazalgette and the Cleansing of the Victorian Metropolis* (Stroud: Sutton, 2007), pp.79-80.

13. Ibid, pp.77-103.

14 Ibid, p.86-8.

15. Ibid, p.90-1.

16. Michael Baker, *The Samuel Bakers, Tradesmen of Kent in the 18th and 19th*

*Centuries*, (Bristol: Michael Baker, 2009).

17. Stephen Halliday, *The Great Stink of London. Sir Joseph Bazalgette and the Cleansing of the Victorian Metropolis* (Stroud: Sutton, 2007), p.98.

18. 'Obituary, Sir Joseph William Bazalgette, C.B., 1819-1891,' *Minutes of the Proceedings*, 105, (1891), pp.302-8, www.icevirtuallibrary.com/content/article/10.1680/imotp.1891.20493 [2014].

19. *The Times*, 24 July 24 1849.

20. Metropolitan Board of Works, *Chelsea Embankment*, (London: Standidge and Co., 1874), pp.7-8.

21. Amanda J. Thomas, *The Lambeth Cholera Outbreak of 1848-1849: The Setting, Causes, Course and Aftermath of an Epidemic in London,* (Jefferson, North Carolina: McFarland & Co., 2009), p.217.

22. Stephen Halliday, *The Great Stink of London. Sir Joseph Bazalgette and the Cleansing of the Victorian Metropolis* (Stroud: Sutton, 2007), p.159.

23. Metropolitan Board of Works, *Chelsea Embankment*, (London: Standidge and Co., 1874), p.10.

24. Minutes of the Proceedings, Vol. 105, Issue 1891, 1 January 1891, Institute of Civil Engineers, (www.icevirtuallibrary.com/content/article/10.1680/imotp.1891.20493), pages 302 –308.

25. Ibid.

26. Ibid, and *Morning Post*, 17 March 1891 (Accessed via Findmypast www.finmypast.co.uk).

27. Thames Water, www.thameswater.co.uk/about-us/10092.htm [2014].

**Chapter 9 Cholera Returns**

1. Sarah Searight, (2003), 'The Charting of the Red Sea,' *History Today*, Vol. 53, Issue 3, www.historytoday.com/sarah-searight/charting-red-sea [2014].

2. Dr Andrew Ashbee, 'In Search of Thomas Fletcher Waghorn (1800-1850),' (*The Clock Tower*, Issue 6, May 2007, The Friends of Medway Archives and Local Studies Centre, www.foma-lsc.org).

3. Sharon Poole and Andrew Sassoli Walker, *P&O Cruises: Celebrating 175 Years of Heritage*, (Stroud: Amberley Publishing Limited, 2013).

4. J. N. Hays, *Epidemics and Pandemics: Their Impacts on Human History*, (ABC-CLIO, 2005), pp.267-8.

5. *The Times*, 27 September 1865.

6. *The Times,* 1 November 1865.

7. *The Times,* 6 November 1866.

8. *The Times* 4, May 1866.

9. *The Times*, 11 June 1866.

10. Amanda J. Thomas, *The Lambeth Cholera Outbreak of 1848-1849: The Setting, Causes, Course and Aftermath of an Epidemic in London,* (Jefferson, North Carolina: McFarland & Co., 2009), p.164.

11. Edmund A. Parkes, *Eighth and Ninth Reports of the Medical Officer of the Privy Council (1866, 1876), (J. roy. Army med. Cps.* 1976 122, George Rosen, M.D., Ph.D, *Edmund A. Parkes In The Development Of Hygiene*, Yale University, New Haven, Connecticut; http://jramc.bmj.com) pp.187-191.

12. Edmund Parkes, (1872), *The British and Foreign Medico-Chirurgical Review*, pp. 67-9,

https://archive.org/stream/britishforeignme50londuoft/britishforeignme50londuoft_djvu.txt [2014].

13. Michael Dunnill, *Dr William Budd, Bristol's most famous physician*, (Bristol: Redcliffe, 2006), pp.57-8.

14. Ibid, pp.59-61.

15. Ibid, pp.97-9.

16. *The Times*, 2 May 1866.

17. *The Times*, 31 October 1866.

18. *The Times*, 6 June 1866.

19. *The Times*, 19 July 1866.

20. *Falkirk Herald*, 19 July 1866.

21. William Farr, *Report on the cholera epidemic of 1866 in England. Supplement to the twenty-ninth annual report of the Registrar-General of Births, Deaths, and Marriages in England*, (London: Eyre and Spottiswoode, 1868), p.111.

22. Ibid, p.114.

23. Ibid, p.115.

24. Ibid.

25. Ibid.

26. Ibid, p.121.

27. Ibid, p.105.

28. Arthur Shadwell, *The London Water Supply*, (London: Longmans, Green, and Co, 1899), p.231.

29. William Farr, *Report on the cholera epidemic of 1866 in England. Supplement to the twenty-ninth annual report of the Registrar-General of Births, Deaths, and Marriages in England*, (London: Eyre and Spottiswoode, 1868), p.117.

30. Ibid, p.119.

31. Ibid, p.121 and 126.

32. Ibid, p.127.

33. Ibid, p.143.

34. William Farr, *Report on the cholera epidemic of 1866 in England. Supplement to the twenty-ninth annual report of the Registrar-General of Births, Deaths, and Marriages in England*, (London: Eyre and Spottiswoode, 1868), Appendix, pp.1 and 5.

35. John M. Eyler, (1973), 'William Farr on the Cholera: The Sanitarian's Disease Theory and the Statistician's Method,' *Journal of the History of Medicine*, pp.95-7, www.medicine.mcgill.ca/epidemiology/hanley/temp/material/SnowCholera/EyleronWilliamFarrCholera.pdf [2014].

36. Ibid.

37. Stephen Halliday, *The Great Stink of London. Sir Joseph Bazalgette and the Cleansing of the Victorian Metropolis* (Stroud: Sutton, 2007), p.141.

38. *The Times*, 11 August 1866.

39. W. H. Michael, *The Sanitary Acts: Comprising the Sewage Utilization Act, 1865, and the Sanitary Act, 1866* , (London: H.Sweet, 1867), p.97.

40. A. J. Ley, *A History of Building Control in England and Wales 1840-1990*, (RICS Books, 2000), pp.62-8.

41. *Public Health Act, 1875*, www.legislation.gov.uk/ukpga/Vict/38-39/55/contents/enacted [2014].

42. Ibid.

43. *The Times*, 12 December 1877.
44. Stephen Halliday, *The Great Stink of London. Sir Joseph Bazalgette and the Cleansing of the Victorian Metropolis* (Stroud, Glos.: Sutton, 2007), p.103.
45. 'SS *Princess Alice*,' *Alsbury Family History*, www.alsbury.co.uk/princess alice/alice0.htm [2014].
46. Ibid.
47. Ibid.
48. *The Times*, 28 September 1878.
49. Ibid.
50. *The Times*, 25 December 1878.
51. *The Times*, 12 September 1878.
52. Stephen Halliday, *The Great Stink of London. Sir Joseph Bazalgette and the Cleansing of the Victorian Metropolis* (Stroud, Glos.: Sutton, 2007), p.103.
53. *The Times*, 30 October 1878.
54. *The Times*, 5 October 1878.
55. 'SS *Princess Alice*,' *Alsbury Family History*, www.alsbury.co.uk/princessalice /alice0.htm, [2014].
56. *The Times*, 5 October 1878.
57. *The Times*, 3 December 1878.
58. *The Times*, 25 November 1878.
59. *The Times*, 18 October 1878.
60. Stephen Halliday, *The Great Stink of London. Sir Joseph Bazalgette and the Cleansing of the Victorian Metropolis* (Stroud: Sutton, 2007), p.106.

**Chapter 10 A Modern Disease**
1. Norman Longmate, *King Cholera. The Biography of a Disease,* (London: Hamish Hamilton, 1966), p. 223.
2. Stephen Halliday, *The Great Stink of London. Sir Joseph Bazalgette and the Cleansing of the Victorian Metropolis* (Stroud: Sutton, 2007), p.143.
3. John G. Avery, *The Cholera Years. An Account of the Cholera Outbreaks in our Ports, Towns and Villages* (Southampton: Beech Books, 2001), p.106.
4. Amanda J. Thomas, *The Lambeth Cholera Outbreak of 1848-1849: The Setting, Causes, Course and Aftermath of an Epidemic in London,* (Jefferson, North Carolina: McFarland & Co., 2009), p.215.
5. Ian Jones, (2014), *The evolution of the cholera vaccine* www.icddrb.org/media-centre/ feature/the-evolution-of-the-oral-cholera-vaccine [2015].
6. Stop Cholera, (2015), www.stopcholera.org [2015].
7. Professor David A. Sack, MD, 5 December 2014
8. Wellcome Trust Sanger Institute, (2014), www.sanger.ac.uk [2014].
9. Professor Nicholas Thomson, Principal Scientist, Bacterial Genomics, Wellcome Trust Sanger Institute, 17 October 2014, (unpublished).
10. Stop Cholera, (2015), www.stopcholera.org [2015].
11. Sandra Moore, et al., (2014), 'Widespread epidemic cholera due to a restricted subset of *Vibrio cholerae* clones,' *Clinical Microbiology and Infection,* pp.373-9, www.ncbi.nlm.nih.gov/pubmed/24575898 [2014].
12. Ibid.
13. Brian Owens, (2011), 'Genomics reveals cholera's travel history,' *Nature News Blog*;

http://blogs.nature.com/news/2011/08/genomics_reveals_choleras_trav.html [2014].

14. Sandra Moore, et al., (2014), 'Widespread epidemic cholera due to a restricted subset of *Vibrio cholerae* clones,' *Clinical Microbiology and Infection,* pp.373-9, www.ncbi.nlm.nih.gov/pubmed/24575898 [2014].

15. Ankur Mutreja, et al, (2011), 'Evidence for Several Waves of Global Transmission in the Seventh Cholera Pandemic,' *Nature,* 477, pp.462-5, www.nature.com/nature/journal/v477/n7365/full/nature10392.html [2014].

16. European Commission Humanitarian Aid Department, *Haiti - Cholera (ECHO Daily Flash, 16 January 2015),* http://reliefweb.int/report/haiti/haiti-cholera-echo-daily-flash-16-january-2015 [2015].

17. UCLA Department of Epidemiology, School of Public Health, John Snow, www.ph.ucla.edu [2014].

18. Dr Ralph Frerichs, Professor Emeritus at the Department of Epidemiology, *UCLA (University of California, Los Angeles)* School of Public Health, 29 June 2012; adapted June 2104, (unpublished).

19. Dr Rita Colwell, *Climate Change, Oceans and Infectious Disease: Cholera Pandemics as a Model*, (Annual Conference of the Society of General Microbiology, April 2014).

20. Ibid.

21. Ibid.

22. Ibid

23. Ibid.

24. Ibid.

# Bibliography

**ARCHIVAL SOURCES**
Ancestry
ARC Archaeological Resource Centre, York
British Library
City of Westminster Archives Centre, London
Findmypast.co.uk
General Register Office, England
John Snow Society
King's College London, Archives and Corporate Records Services, Information
    Services and Systems, London
Lambeth Archives Department, Lambeth, London.
London Metropolitan Archives, London.
London School of Hygiene and Tropical Medicine
The Royal College of Physicians
The Royal College of Surgeons of England
Times Digital Archive
St. Bartholomew's Hospital, Archives and Museum, London
Tyne and Wear Archives
Wellcome Library
Wellcome Trust Sanger Institute
World Health Organization
York Museums Trust

**BOOKS**
Alderson, James, *A Brief Outline of the History and Progress of Cholera at Hull*,
    (London: Longman, Rees, Orme, Brown, Green & Longman, 1832).
Alexander, Marc, *The Sutton Companion to the Folklore, Myths and Customs of
    Britain*, (Stroud, Glos.: The History Press, 2005).
Anon., *The Glass Industry of Tyne and Wear; Part One: Glassmaking on Wearside*,
    (Tyne and Wear County Council (Museums), 1979; L/PA/146).
Arnold, Catharine, *Necropolis: London and Its Dead*, (London: Simon & Schuster, 2006).
Arnold, Matthew, *Culture and Anarchy*, (Oxford: Oxford University Press, 2009).
Atkinson Hobson, John, *Problems of Poverty: and Inquiry into the Industrial Condition
    of the Poor*, (Memphis: General Books, 2012).
Avery, John G., *The Cholera Years. An Account of the Cholera Outbreaks in our Ports,
    Towns and Villages* (Southampton: Beech Books, 2001).
Baker, Michael, *The Samuel Bakers, Tradesmen of Kent in the 18th and 19th Centuries*,
    (Bristol: Michael Baker, 2009).
Baly, William and Gull, William Withey, *Report on the Nature and Import of Certain
    Microscopic Bodies Found in the Intestinal Discharges of Cholera: Presented to the
    Cholera Committee of the Royal College of Physicians...by Their Sub-committee, on*

*the 17th October, 1849*, Cholera Committee, Royal College of Physicians (London: John Churchill, 1849).

Barnard, Sylvia M., *To Prove I'm Not Forgot: Living and Dying in a Victorian City*, (Manchester University Press, 1990).

Barrett, Ron, Armelagos, George J., *An Unnatural History of Emerging Infections*, (New York: Oxford University Press, 2013).

Barton, Nicholas, *The Lost Rivers of London*, (London: Historical Publications Ltd, 2005).

Behagg, Clive, *Labour and Reform, Working-Class Movements 1815-1914*, (London: Hodder and Stoughton, 1991).

Besant, Walter, *London in the Nineteenth Century*. (London: Forgotten Books, 2013; originally published 1909).

Billington, Mike, *Using the Building Regulations: Administrative Procedures*, (London: Routledge, 2006).

Blaine, Gilbert, *A Warning to the British Public Against the Alarming Approach of the Indian cholera and the History of the Epidemic Cholera of India, from its first appearance in the year 1817, to 1831, and the dreadful ravages it has committed, with the dates of its first appearance in the different provinces;* (London: Burgess and Hill, 1831).

Boisseau, François Gabriel, *A Treatise on Cholera Morbus: Or, Researches on the Symptoms, Nature, and Treatment of the Disease: And on the Different Means of Avoiding it*, (New York: Collins & Co, 1832).

Brown, Kevin, *Poxed & Scurvied: The Story of Sickness and Health at Sea*, (Barnsley: Seaforth Publishing, 2011).

Budd, William, *Malignant Cholera: its cause, mode of propagation, and prevention, (International Journal of Epidemiology* 2013;42:1567–1575, doi:10.1093/ije/dyt204, (http://ije.oxfordjournals.org/content/42/6/1567.short) pp.1567-1574.
William Budd, *Malignant Cholera: its cause, mode of propagation, and prevention, (London: Churchill, 1849).*

Burch, Druin, *Digging up the Dead, Uncovering the Life and Times of an Extraordinary Surgeon*, (London: Vintage, 2007).

Burton, Anthony, *Canal 250. The Story of Britain's Canals*, (Stroud: The History Press, 2011).

Burton, Anthony, *The Canal Builders*, (Gloucestershire: Tempus, 2005).

Chadwick, Edwin, *Report on the Sanitary Condition of the Labouring Population of Great Britain. A Supplementary Report On the Results of a Special Inquiry into the Practice of Interment in Towns*, (London: W. Clowes, 1843).

Checkland, SG and EAO, *The Poor Law Report of 1834*, (Harmondsworth: Penguin Books, 1974).

Clanny, William Reid, *Hyperanthraxis; Or, the Cholera of Sunderland*, (London: Whittaker, Treacher and Arnott, 1832).

Cook, Chris, *The Routledge Companion to Britain in the Nineteenth Century, 1815-1914*, (London: Routledge, 2005).

Cunningham Glen, Dr. William, *The Nuisances Removal and Diseases Prevention Acts, 1848 & 1849: (11 & 12 Vict. Cap. 123 ; 12 & 13 Vict. Cap. 111) with Practical Notes and Appendix containing the Directions and Regulations of the General Board of Health, with Index*, (Third Edition, London: Shaw and Sons, 1849).

# BIBLIOGRAPHY

Defoe, Daniel, *A Journal of the Plague Year. Being Observations or Memorials of the Most Remarkable Occurrences, as well Publick as Private, which Happened in London During the Great Visitation in 1665. Written by a Citizen who Continued all the While in London, Never Made Publick Before,* (London: George Routledge and Sons, 1886).

Dobson, Mary, *Disease: The Extraordinary Stories Behind History's Deadliest Killers,* (London: Quercus, 2007).

Dodsworth, Roger, *Glass and Glassmaking,* (Buckinghamshire: Shire Publications Ltd, 2003).

Drasar, B.S, Forrest, B.D., *Cholera and the Ecology of* Vibrio cholerae, (London: Chapman & Hall, 1996).

Dunnill, Michael, *Dr William Budd, Bristol's most famous physician,* (Bristol: Redcliffe, 2006).

Durey, M., *The First Spasmodic Cholera Epidemic in York, 1832* (York: St Anthony's Press, 1974).

Dutt, Romesh Chunder, *The Economic History of India in the Victorian Age: From the Accession of Queen Victoria in 1837 to the Commencement of the Twentieth Century,* (London: Routledge, 2013).

Ekelund, Robert B. Price, Edward O., *The Economics of Edwin Chadwick: Incentives Matter,* (Cheltenham: Edward Elgar Publishing, 2012).

Engels, Friedrich, *The Condition of the Working Class in England,* (London: Penguin Classics, 2005).

Farr, William, *Report on the cholera epidemic of 1866 in England. Supplement to the twenty-ninth annual report of the Registrar-General of Births, Deaths, and Marriages in England,* (London: Eyre and Spottiswoode, 1868).

Faruque, Shah M. G., Nair, Balakrish, *Vibrio Cholerae: Genomics and Molecular Biology,* (Horizon Scientific Press, 2008).

Flanders, Judith, *The Victorian City: Everyday Life in Dickens' London,* (London: Atlantic Books, 2012).

Flinn, M.W., *Introduction; Report on The Sanitary Condition of the Labouring Population of Great Britain* by Edwin Chadwick, 1842; (Edinburgh University Press, 1965).

Flood, Raymond, Rice, Adrian, Wilson, Robin, *Mathematics in Victorian Britain,* (Oxford: Oxford University Press, 2011).

Friedman, Daniel J., Gibson Parrish, Edward L. R., *Health Statistics: Shaping Policy and Practice to Improve the Population's Health,* (Oxford: Oxford University Press, 2005).

Gaulter, Henry, The Origin and Progress of the Malignant Cholera in Manchester, (Memphis: General Books, 2012).

Gibbons, David, *The Metropolitan Buildings Act. 7th & 8th. Vict. Cap. 84. With Notes and an Index,* (London: Weale, 1844).

Gladstone, David, and Finer, Samuel Edward, *Edwin Chadwick: Nineteenth-century Social Reform,* (London: Routledge, 1997).

Glyde, John, *The Moral, Social and religious Condition of Ipswich in the Middle of the Nineteenth Century,* (Ipswich: J.M. Burton & Co.,1850; BiblioLife, 2009).

Halliday, Stephen, *The Great Stink of London. Sir Joseph Bazalgette and the Cleansing of the Victorian Metropolis* (Stroud: Sutton, 2007).

231

Halliday, Stephen, *The War against Disease in Victorian England. The Great Filth*, (Stroud: Sutton, 2007).

Hamlin, Christopher, *Cholera: The Biography*, (New York: Oxford University Press, 2009).

Hamlin, Christopher, *Public Health and Social Justice in the Age of Chadwick: Britain, 1800-1854*, (Cambridge University Press, 1998).

Hays, J. N., *Epidemics and Pandemics: Their Impacts on Human History*, (ABC-CLIO, 2005).

Higginbotham, Peter, (2014), *The Lancet Reports on Metropolitan Workhouse Infirmaries, 1865-66: Camberwell*, www.workhouses.org.uk/Lancet/Camberwell.shtml [2014].

Hobson, John Atkinson, *Problems of Poverty: An Inquiry Into the Industrial Condition of the Poor*, (RareBooksClub.com, 2012).

Hodgkinson, Ruth G., *The Origins of the National Health Service: the medical services of the new Poor Law, 1834-1871*, (California: University of California Press, California, 1967).

Hollingshead, John, *Ragged London in 1861*, (London: Smith, Elder and Co., 1861).

Koch, Tom, *Disease Maps, Epidemics on the Ground*, (University of Chicago Press, 2011).

Labbé, Ronald G., García, Santos, *Guide to Foodborne Pathogens*, (Chichester: Wiley-Blackwell, 2013).

Lane, Joan, *A Social History of Medicine: Health, Healing and Disease in England, 1750-1950*, (London: Routledge, 2012).

Lankester, Edwin, *Cholera: what is it? And How to Prevent it* (1866; RareBooksClub.com, 2012).

Laxton, William, *The Civil Engineer and Architect's Journal, Volume 13*, (Pub. for the proprietor, 1850).

Ley, A. J., *A History of Building Control in England and Wales 1840-1990*, (RICS Books, 2000).

Longmate, Norman, *King Cholera. The Biography of a Disease*, (London: Hamish Hamilton, 1966).

Malthus, T.R., *An Essay on the Principle of Population*, (Oxford: Oxford University Press, 2008).

McLean, David, *Public Health and Politics in the Age of Reform*, (London: I.B. Tauris & Co. Ltd., 2006).

Metropolitan Board of Works, *Chelsea Embankment*, (London: Standidge and Co., 1874).

Michael, W. H, *The Sanitary Acts: Comprising the Sewage Utilization Act, 1865, and the Sanitary Act, 1866*, (London: 1867).

Midwinter, Eric C., *Social Administration in Lancashire, 1830-1860: Poor Law, Public Health and Police*, (Manchester University Press, 1969).

Morabia, Alfredo, *A History of Epidemiologic Methods and Concepts*, (Springer Science & Business Media, 2004).

Needham, J P., *Facts and observations relative to the disease commonly called cholera, as it has recently prevailed in the city of York*, (London: Longman, Rees, Orme, Brown, Green, and Co, 1833).

Newton, John Frank, *The Return to Nature: or, A defence of the vegetable regimen; with some account of an experiment made during the last three or four years in the author's family, Volume 6*, (London: T. Cadell and W. Davies, 1811).

# BIBLIOGRAPHY

Nicholson, Adam, *Gentry. Six Hundred Years of a Peculiarly English Class*, (London: Harper Press, 2011).

Northend, J.W., *The history of the cholera epidemic of 1832 in Sheffield*, (Sheffield: John Stokes, 1921).

Pelling, Margaret, *Cholera, Fever and English Medicine, 1825-1865*, (Oxford: Oxford University Press, 1978).

Poole, Sharon and Sassoli Walker, Andrew, *P&O Cruises: Celebrating 175 Years of Heritage*, (Stroud: Amberley Publishing Limited, 2013).

Pooley, Colin, Turnbull, Jean, *Migration and Mobility in Britain Since the 18th Century*, (London: Routledge, 2003).

Porter, Dorothy, *Health, Civilization and the State: A History of Public Health from Ancient to Modern Times*, (London: Routledge, 1999).

Rees, Rosemary, *Poverty and Public Health, 1815-1948*, (Oxford: Heinemann, 2001).

Richetti, John *The Life of Daniel Defoe: A Critical Biography*, (Chichester: Wiley-Blackwell, 2008).

Robson, William A., *The Government and Misgovernment of London*, (London: Routledge, 2013).

Rodger, Richard, *Housing in Urban Britain 1780-1914*, (Cambridge University Press, 1995).

Rosen, George, *A History of Public Health*, (Baltimore, Maryland: John Hopkins University Press, 1993).

Sedgwick, W. T., *Principles of sanitary science and the public health with special reference to the causation and prevention of infectious diseases*, (New York: The Macmillan Company, 1902).

Shadwell, Arthur, *The London Water Supply*, (London: Longmans, Green, and Co., 1899).

Shapter, Thomas, *The History of the Cholera in Exeter in 1832*, (Wakefield and London: S.R. Publishers Ltd., 1971).

Sherwood, Tim, *The Steamboat Revolution: London's First Steamships* (Gloucestershire, Tempus, 2007).

Simon, Dr. John, *Report on the last two Cholera-Epidemics of London, as affected by the consumption of impure water.* (George E. Eyre and William Spottiswood, 1856).

Sloane, Barney, *The Black Death in London*, (Stroud: The History Press, 2011).

Snow, John, *On the Mode of Communication of Cholera*, (London: John Churchill, 1855).

Sturgess, R.W., *The Great Age of Industry in the North East*, (Durham County Local History Society, 1981).

Thackrah, Charles Turner, *Cholera, its Character and Treatment: with Remarks on the Identity of The Indian and English, and a Particular Reference to the Disease as now Existent in Newcastle and its Neighbourhood*, (Leeds: J. Baines & Co., 1832).

Thomas Sydenham, *The Works of Thomas Sydenham, M.D., on Acute and Chronic Diseases: With Their Histories and Modes of Cure*, (Philadelphia: B. & T. Kite, 1809).

Thomas, Amanda J., *The Lambeth Cholera Outbreak of 1848-1849: The Setting, Causes, Course and Aftermath of an Epidemic in London*, (Jefferson, North Carolina: McFarland & Co., 2009).

Thompson, E. P., *The Making of the English Working Class*, (England: Penguin Books, 1991).

Troyer, John, *The Classical Utilitarians: Bentham and Mill,* (Indianapolis: Hackett Publishing, 2003).

Vinten-Johansen, Peter et al, *Cholera, Chloroform, and the Science of Medicine: A Life of John Snow*, (New York: Oxford University Press, 2003).

Walker, George Alfred, *Gatherings from Grave Yards, Particularly Those of London: with a Concise History of the Modes of Interment Among Different Nations, from the Earliest Periods. And a Detail of Dangerous and Fatal Results Produced by the Unwise and Revolting Custom of Inhuming the Dead in the Midst of the Living,* (London: Longman and Co., 1839).

Watts, Duncan, *Tories, Unionists and Conservatives (1815-1914)* (London: Hodder & Stoughton, 2002).

Watts, Duncan, *Whigs, Radicals and Liberals 1815-1914*, (London: Hodder Murray, 2002).

Watts, Sheldon, *Epidemics and History: Disease, Power and Imperialism*, (Newhaven and London: Yale University Press, 1999).

**ARTICLES AND PAPERS**

Ackerknecht, Erwin H., 'Anticontagionism Between 1821 and 1867,' The Fielding H. Garrison Lecture, (*International Journal of Epidemiology*, Vol. 38, Issue 1).

Ali Shafqat Akanda, Jutla, A.S., Gute, D.M., Sack, R.B., Alam, M., Huq, A., Colwell, R.R., Islam, S., (2013),'Population Vulnerability to Biannual Cholera Outbreaks and Associated Macro-Scale Drivers in the Bengal Delta,' *The American Journal of Tropical Medicine and Hygiene*, 89(5), pp.950-9, www.frontiersin.org/profile/publications/23736910, [2014].

Altonen, Brian, '1852 – William Farr's Elevation and Cholera Paper,' *Public Health, Medicine and History,* (http://brianaltonenmph.com/gis/historical-medical-geography/1852-william-farr-elevation-and-cholera [2014].

Anning, S.T., (1969), 'Leeds House of Recovery,' *Medical History*, 13(3), pp.226-236, europepmc.org/articles/PMC1033950/pdf/medhist00138-0018.pdf☐ [2014].

Ashbee, Dr Andrew, (2007), 'In Search of Thomas Fletcher Waghorn (1800-1850),' *The Clock Tower*, Issue 6, www.foma-lsc.org, [2014].

Ashworth Underwood, E., *The History of the 1832 Cholera Epidemic in Yorkshire*, (Proceedings of the Royal Society of Medicine, Vol. XXVIII, 608, 1935).

Bedford, D. Evan, Hartston, William and Drew, Sir Robert, (1976), 'An Early Account of Rheumatic Heart Disease by Joseph Brown (1784-1868),' *Medical History*, 20(1), pp.76-9, http://europepmc.org/articles/PMC1081694/pdf/medhist00112-0080.pdf [2014].

Bell, John, Condie, David Francis, *All the Material Facts in the History of Epidemic Cholera: Being a Report of the College of Physicians of Philadelphia, to the Board of Health: and a Full Account of the Causes, Post Mortem Appearances, and Treatment of the Disease,* (Philadelphia: Thomas Desilver, jun., 1832).

Bennish, Michael L., 'Cholera: Pathophysiology, Clinical Features and Treatment,' in I. Kaye Wachsmuth, Paul A. Blake, and Ørjan Olsvik, eds., Vibrio cholerae *and Cholera. Molecular to Global Perspectives* (Washington DC: American Society for Microbiology, 1994).

Billing, Archibald, M.D., A.M., F.R.S., 'On The Treatment of Asiatic Cholera,' 2d ed., revised (London: S. Highley, 1848), from William Baly, *Reports on Epidemic Cholera: Drawn up at the desire of the Cholera Committee of the Royal College of*

# BIBLIOGRAPHY

*Physicians*, Cholera Committee, Royal College of Physicians (London: J. Churchill, 1854), Ref. SLTr80.

Blokesch, Melanie, 'The Lifestyle of *Vibrio cholerae* Fosters Gene Transfers,' (*Microbe*, Vol. 9, No. 2, 2014).

Bos et al, 'A draft genome of Yersinia pestis from victims of the Black Death,' (Nature 478, (27 October 2011); doi:10.1038/nature10549).

Parkes, E.A., (1855), 'Review of Snow's Mode of Communication of Cholera,' British and Foreign Medical Review, http://johnsnow.matrix.msu.edu/work.php ?id=15-78-C1[2014].

Budd, William, (1867), 'Asiatic Cholera in Bristol in 1866,' *British Medical Journal*, 1(328) , pp.413–420, www.ncbi.nlm.nih.gov/pmc/articles/PMC2309505, [2014].

Burns, J. H., *Happiness and Utility: Jeremy Bentham's Equation*, www.utilitarianism. com/jeremy-bentham/greatest-happiness.pdf, [2014]..

Cabuguason, Gleisel, 'The Microbiology of the *Vibrio cholerae Bacterium*,' http://cosmos.ucdavis.edu/archives/2007/cluster7/cabuguason_gleisel.pdf [2015].

Cooney, Catherine M., (2012), 'Rita Colwell: Keeping Her Aim on Cholera,' *Earthzine* www.earthzine.org/2012/11/28/rita-colwell-keeping-her-aim-on-cholera, [2014].

Cooper, Edmund, *Report to the Metropolitan Commission of Sewers on the house-drainage in St. James, Westminster during the recent cholera outbreak*, 22 Sep 1854, (London Metropolitan Archives).

Curle, B. R., (1969), 'Mr Drouet's Establishment at Tooting: an Essay in Victorian Child Welfare,' *Surrey Archaeological Collections,* 66, http://archaeology dataservice. ac.uk/archiveDS/archiveDownload?t=arch-379-1/dissemination/pdf/vol _66/surreyac066_087-098_curle.pdf [2014].

Curtis, V., S. Cairncross, S., (2003), 'Effect of washing hand with soap on diarrhoea risk in the community: a systematic review,' The *Lancet, Infectious Diseases*, 3(5), pp. 275-81 (Abstract), http://www.ncbi.nlm.nih.gov/pubmed/12726975 [2014].

Curtis, V., Schmidt, W., Luby, S., Florez, R., Touré, O., Biran, A.,(2011), 'Hygiene: new hopes, new horizons,' The *Lancet, Infectious Diseases*, 11(4), pp. 312-21, www.ncbi. nlm.nih.gov/pubmed/21453872 [2014].

Devault, Alison M., et al, (2014), 'Second-Pandemic Strain of *Vibrio cholerae* from the Philadelphia Cholera Outbreak of 1849,' *The New England Journal of Medicine*, 370, pp.344-40, www.nejm.org/doi/full/10.1056/NEJMoa1308663, [2014].

Dickens, Charles, (1849), 'The Paradise at Tooting,' *The Examiner,* www.workhouses. org.uk/Drouet/Examiner1.shtml

Dickens, Charles, Jr., (1879), *Dickens's Dictionary of London*, www.victorianlondon. org/publications/dictionary.htm, [2014].

Dueker, M. Elias, O'Mullan, Gregory D., (2014), 'Aeration remediation of a polluted waterway increases near-surface coarse and culturable microbial aerosols,' *Science of the Total Environment*, 478.

Dunn, P.M., (2002), 'Perinatal lessons from the past; Dr William Farr of Shropshire (1807– 1883): obstetric mortality and training,' (*Archives of Disease in Childhood, Fetal & Neonatal Edition,* 87, http://fn.bmj.com/content/87/1/F67.full, [2014].

Eyler, John M., (1973), 'William Farr on the Cholera: The Sanitarian's Disease Theory and the Statistician's Method,' *Journal of the History of Medicine,* www.medicine.mcgill.ca/epidemiology/hanley/temp/material/SnowCholera/ EyleronWilliamFarrCholera.pdf [2014].

Faruque, S.M., Naser, I.B., Islam, M.J., Faruque, A.S., Ghosh, A.N., Nair, G.B., Sack, D.A., Mekalanos, J.J., (2005), 'Seasonal epidemics of cholera inversely correlate with the prevalence of environmental cholera phages,' *Proceedings of the National Academy of Sciences of the United States of America*, 102 (5), pp. 1702-7, www.ncbi.nlm.nih.gov/pubmed/15653771 [2014].

Fisher, Pam 'Houses for the Dead: The Provision of Mortuaries in London, 1843–1889,' (*The London Journal*, Vol. 34 No. 1, March, 2009).

Galbraith, Spence. *Dr. John Snow (1813-1858) - His Early Years*, (Royal Institute of Public Health, 2002), (www.ph.ucla.edu/epi/snow.html).

Grimes, D.J., Ford, T.E., Colwell, R.R., Baker-Austin, C., Martinez-Urtaza, J., Subramaniam, A., Capone, D.G., (2014), 'Viewing Marine Bacteria, Their Activity and Response to Environmental Drivers from Orbit: Satellite Remote Sensing of Bacteria,' Microbial Ecology, 67 93), pp.489-500, www.frontiersin.org/profile/publications/24209888, [2014].

Haley, B.J., Choi, S.Y., Grim, C.J., Onifade, T.J., Cinar, H.N., Tall, B.D., Taviani, E., Hasan, N.A., Abdullah, A.H., Carter, L., Sahu, S.N., Kothary, M.H., Chen, A., Baker, R., Hutchinson, R., Blackmore, C., Cebula, T.A., Huq, A., Colwell, R.R.,(2014), 'Genomic and Phenotypic Characterization of *Vibrio cholerae* Non-O1 Isolates from a US Gulf Coast Cholera Outbreak,' *PLoS One*, 9(4) , www.ncbi.nlm.nih.gov/pubmed/24699521

Hamlin, Christopher, 'Public Health Then and Now. Could You Starve to Death in England in 1839? The Chadwick-Farr Controversy and the Loss of the "Social" in Public Health,' (*American Journal of Public Health*, June 1995, Vol. 85, No. 6).

Jefferies, Julie, *Focus On, People and Migration The UK population: past, present and future*, (Office for National Statistics, 2005).

Jensen, Mark A., Faruque, Shah M., Mekalanos, John J., and Levin Bruce R., (2006), 'Modeling the role of bacteriophage in the control of cholera outbreaks,' *Proceedings of the National Academy of Sciences of the United States of America*, 103 (12), pp.4652-4657, www.pnas.org/content/103/12/4652.abstract [2014].

Johnson, James, *The Medico-Chirurgical Review and Journal of Practical Medicine* Vol. 20, (S. Highley, 1832).

Jutla, A., Whitcombe, E., Hasan, N., Haley, B., Akanda, A., Huq, A., Alam, M., Sack, R.B., Colwell, R., (2013), 'Environmental Factors Influencing Epidemic Cholera,' *The American Journal of Tropical Medicine and Hygiene*, June, 89(3), pp597-607, www.ncbi.nlm.nih.gov/pubmed/23897993 [2014].

Kershaw, Ian, (1973), 'The Great Famine And Agrarian Crisis In England 1315-1322,' *Past and Present*, 59 (1), http://links.jstor.org, [2014].

Kiiru, John, Mutreja, Ankur, Mohamed, Ahmed Abade, Kimani, Racheal W., Mwituria, Joyce, Onsare Sanaya, Robert, Muyodi, Jane, Revathi, Gunturu, Parkhill, Julian, Thomson, Nicholas, Dougan, Gordon, Kariuki. Samuel, (2013), 'A Study on the Geophylogeny of Clinical and Environmental *Vibrio cholerae* in Kenya,' PLoS One, DOI: 10.1371, www.plosone.org/article/info:doi/10.1371/journal.pone.0074829, [2014].

Klose K.E., Mekalanos, J.J., (1998), 'Distinct roles of an alternative sigma factor during both free-swimming and colonizing phases of the *Vibrio cholerae* pathogenic cycle,' *Molecular Microbiology*, 28(3), pp.501-20, www.ncbi.nlm.nih.gov/pubmed/9632254, [2014].

Koch, Tom, Denike, Kenneth, (2009), 'Crediting his critics' concerns: Remaking John Snow's map of Broad Street cholera, 1854,' *Social Science & Medicine,* 69(8) pp.1246–1251, www.elsevier.com, [2014].

Macnalty, Arthur S., *British Medical Journal,* 25 Sep 1965.

Manby, E., *Dissertation, with Practical Remarks, on Cholera Morbus,* (London: Burgess and Hill, 1831), from William Baly, *Reports on Epidemic Cholera: Drawn up at the desire of the Cholera Committee of the Royal College of Physicians,* Cholera Committee, Royal College of Physicians (London: J. Churchill, 1854), Ref. SLTr80.

Miller, Andrew, *The Rise And Progress Of Coatbridge And Surrounding Neighbourhood, Dundyvan Iron Works, Glasgow 1864,* www.scottishmining.co.uk/415.html [2014].

Moore, Sandra, Thomson, Nicholas, Mutreja, Ankur, and Piarroux, Renaud, (2011), 'Cholera Pandemic's Source Discovered,' www.sanger.ac.uk/about/press/2011/110824.html [2014].

Moore, Sandra, Thomson, Nicholas, Mutreja, Ankur, and Piarroux, Renaud, (2014), 'Widespread epidemic cholera due to *Vibrio cholerae* clones,' *Clinical Microbiology and Infection,* 20 (5), pp.373-9, www.ncbi.nlm.nih.gov/pubmed/24575898 [2014].

Morris, John S, (2007), 'Sir Henry Halford, president of the Royal College of Physicians, with a note on his involvement in the exhumation of King Charles I,' Postgrad Medical Journal, 83(980) , pp.431–433, www.ncbi.nlm.nih.gov/pmc/articles/PMC2600044 [2014].

Morris, R. J., (1977), 'Cholera 1832 – The Social Response to An Epidemic,' *Medical History,* 21(3), p.336, www.ph.ucla.edu/epi/snow/morris/morris_lessons_a.html, [2014].

Mutreja, Ankur Kim, Dong Wook, Thomson, Nicholas R., Connor, Thomas R., Lee, Je Hee, Kariuki, Samuel, Croucher, Nicholas J., Choi, Seon Young, Harris, Simon R., Lebens, Michael, Niyogi, Swapan Kumar, Kim, Eun Jin, Ramamurthy, T., Chun, Jongsik, Wood, James L. N., Clemens, John D., Czerkinsky, Cecil, Nair, G. Balakrish, Holmgren, Jan, Parkhill, Julian, Dougan, Gordon. (2011), 'Evidence for Several Waves of Global Transmission in the Seventh Cholera Pandemic,' *Nature,* doi:10.1038/nature10392.

Olsen, G.N, Rennie, Foster, Fresh, T., MEPAS, Newlands, J., (1998) 'Liverpool's drainage history: seventeenth century to MEPAS,' *Municipal Engineer,* 121, (2), 67-77. www.icevirtuallibrary.com/content/article/10.1680/imuen.1997.29487 [2014]

Owens, Brian, (2011), 'Genomics reveals cholera's travel history,' *Nature News Blog;* http://blogs.nature.com/news/2011/08/genomics_reveals_choleras_trav.html, [2014].

Parkes, Edmund, *The British and Foreign Medico-Chirurgical Review,* Quarterly Journal, Practical Medicine And Surgery. Vol. L., July - October, 1872 (London: J. & A. Churchill, 1872.), https://archive.org/stream/britishforeignme50londuoft/britishforeignme50 londuoft_djvu.txt [2014].

Public Health Act, 1875, www.legislation.gov.uk/ukpga/Vict/38-39/55/contents/enacted [2014].

Simon, Dr John, (1856), *Report on the Last Two Cholera-Epidemics of London, as Affected by the Consumption of Impure Water,* http://johnsnow.matrix.msu.edu/work.php?id=15-78-7F [2014].

# CHOLERA

Rashid, A., Haley, B.J., Rajabov, M., Ahmadova, S., Gurbanov, S., Colwell, R.R., Huq, A., (2013), 'Detection of Vibrio cholerae in environmental waters including drinking water reservoirs of Azerbaijan,' *Environmental Microbiology Reports*, 5(1), pp30-8, www.frontiersin.org/profile/publications/23514031 [2014].

Rhodes, Glenn, Richardson, Hollian, Hermon-Taylor, John, Weightman, Andrew, Higham, Andrew, and Pickup Roger, (2014), '*Mycobacterium avium* Subspecies *paratuberculosis*: Human Exposure through Environmental and Domestic Aerosols,' *Pathogens*, 3(3), pp.577-595, www.mdpi.com/2076-0817/3/3/577 [2014].

Roberts, Andrew, (1991), *England's Poor Law Commissioners and the Trade in Pauper Lunacy, 1834-1847*, http://studymore.org.uk/mott.htm [2014].

Sack, David A., Sack, R Bradley, Balakrish Nair, G., Siddique, A.K., (2004), 'Cholera,' *The Lancet*, 363, www.ph.ucla.edu/epi/snow/lancet363_223_233_2004.pdf, [2014]. McMaster University, *Daily News*, (27 January 2014), 'Scientists Reveal Cause of one of the most Devastating Pandemics in Human History,' *Daily News*, http://dailynews.mcmaster.ca [2014].

Searight, Sarah, (2003), 'The Charting of the Red Sea,' *History Today*, Vol. 53, Issue 3, www.historytoday.com/sarah-searight/charting-red-sea [2014].

Shah, Muhammad Ali, Mutreja, Ankur, Thomson, Nicholas, Baker, Stephen, Parkhill, Julian, Dougan, Gordon, Bokhari, Habib, and Wren, Brendan W., (2014), 'Genomic epidemiology of *Vibrio cholerae* O1 associated with floods, Pakistan, 2010,' *Emerging Infectious Diseases Journal*, 20 (1), http://dx.doi.org/10.3201/eid2001.130428, [2014].

Stephanie J. Snow, (2000), 'John Snow MD (1813-1858). Part II: Becoming a doctor - his medical training and early years of practice,' *Journal of Medical Biography*, 8, www.ph.ucla.edu/epi/snow/jmedbiography8_71_77_2000.pdf [2014].

Snow, Thomas., 'Doctor's teetotal address delivered in 1836.' (*The British Temperance Advocate*, 1888), http://johnsnow.matrix.msu.edu/work.php?id=15-78-1 [2014]. Starr, Cecie, Taggart, Ralph, Evers, Christine, Starr, Lisa, (2008), 'Biology: The Unity and Diversity of Life,' *Cengage Learning*, www.cengagebrain.com [2014].

Tonne, Cathryn, Wilkinson, Paul, (2013) 'Long-term exposure to air pollution is associated with survival following acute coronary syndrome,' *European Heart Journal*, http://eurheartj.oxfordjournals.org/content/early/2013/02/18/eurheartj.ehs480 [2014].

Whitehead M., (2000), 'William Farr's Legacy to the Study of Inadequacies in Health,' *Bulletin of the World Health Organisation*, 78(1), pp.86-87, www.ncbi.nlm.nih.gov/pmc/articles/PMC2560600 [2014].

Zuck, David, *Charles Empson*, David Zuck, *Charles Empson*, http://kora.matrix.msu.edu/files/21/120/15-78-18B-22-Empsonbiogdefin05.pdf [2014]. *The Burial Board Acts of England and Wales*, (London: William Cunningham Glen, Shaw and Sons, 1868,), 16 & 17 Vict. Cap. 134, pp.80-1; https://archive.org/stream/burialboardacts00glengoog/burialboardacts00glengoog_djvu.txt [2014].

Royal College of Surgeons, (2012), *Plarr's Lives of the Fellows Online*, Greenhow, Thomas Michael, http://livesonline.rcseng.ac.uk/biogs/E002048b.htm [2014]. 'Sackville Street,' Survey of London: volumes 31 and 32: St James Westminster, Part 2 (1963), www.british-history.ac.uk/report.aspx?compid=41480, [2014].

Victoria County History, 'How the central settlements of Sunderland grew to become a town,' *Growth of the Town, 1600-1800*, Durham Volume V: Sunderland, www.

victoriacountyhistory.ac.uk/counties/durham/work-in-progress/growth-town-1600-1800 [2014].

World Health Organization, (2003), 'Algae and cyanobacteria in coastal and estuarine waters,' *Guidelines For Safe Recreational Water Environments, Volume 1: Coastal And Fresh Waters;* Chapter 7, www.who.int/water_sanitation_health/bathing/srwe1-chap7.pdf [2014].

## REPORTS AND MINUTES

*General Board of Health Report of the Committee for Scientific Inquiries in Relation to the Cholera-Epidemic of 1854*, (London: Eyre & Spottiswoode, 1855, The John Snow Archive and Research Companion; http://johnsnow.matrix.msu.edu/work.php?id=15-78-BE).

'Metropolitan Sewage Committee Proceedings; *Parliamentary Papers*, 1846: vol. 10. Minutes of the Proceedings,' Vol. 105, Issue 1891, 1 January 1891, Institute of Civil Engineers, www.icevirtuallibrary.com/content/article/10.1680/imotp.1891.20493. [2014]

'Report from His Majesty's Commissioners for Inquiring into the Administration and Practical Operation of the Poor Laws, 1834,' *London Gazette*, 1834.

*Report on the Cholera Outbreak in the Parish of St James, Westminster, during the Autumn of 1854.* Presented to the Vestry by the Cholera Inquiry Committee, July 1855, (London: John. Churchill, 1855, http://johnsnow.matrix.msu.edu/work.php?id=15-78-AA. [2014].

Sutherland, Dr John, *Report of the General Board of Health on the Epidemic Cholera of 1848 &1849* (London: Clowes & Son, 1850).

*Sir John Simon's Medical Officer of Health reports on the* Sanitary Condition of London, *1848-55*, Medical Officer of Health Reports 1848-9.

## NEWSPAPERS AND PERIODICALS

British Newspaper Archive, (www.findmypast.co.uk).

*The Cholera Gazette, Vol. 1-16*, (Memphis: General Books, 2012).

*The Clock Tower*, The Friends Of Medway Archives and Local Studies Centre.

*The Guardian*, (www.theguardian.com).

*Parliamentary Papers, House of Commons and Command*, Vol. 17, (H.M. Stationery Office, 1831).

*Pigot and Co.'s National Commercial Directory of the Whole of Scotland and of The Isle of Man: with a General Alphabetical List of the Nobility, Gentry and Clergy of Scotland* (James Pigot and Co., London, 1837).

*The Pollution of Rivers Commission, Second Report* (London: Her Majesty's Stationery Office, 1867).

*The Quarterly Review, Vol. XLVI, November. 1831 and January 1832*, (London: John Murray, 1832).

*The Times* Digital Archive.

*Wolverhampton Chronicle*, (www.wolverhamptonhistory.org.uk).

## WEBSITES

Alsbury Family History: www.alsbury.co.uk/princessalice/alice0.htm

Ancestry: www.ancestry.co.uk

Internet Archive: https://archive.org

Carnegie Mellon University, Pittsburgh, Department of Philosophy:
  http://caae.phil.cmu.edu/Cavalier
Education Scotland: www.educationscotland.gov.uk
1837.com: www.1837.com/civil-registration
English Heritage: www.english-heritage.org.uk
History of Economic Thought: http://historyofeconomicthought.wikispaces.com
History of Health and Healthcare, Curriculum for Excellence Resource: http://ewds.
  strath.ac.uk/historymedicine/Resources/ByType/MedicalOfficerofHealthReports.aspx
Ice Virtual Library, Institution of Civil Engineers: www.icevirtuallibrary.com
Lancashire Infantry Museum: www.lancashireinfantrymuseum.org.uk
Lambeth Landmark, Lambeth Archives Image Collection: http://landmark.lambeth.gov.uk
Liverpool Picture Book: www.liverpoolpicturebook.com/2012/10/HousingandHealth
  Liverpool.html
Merton Historical Society: www.mertonhistoricalsociety.org.uk
Museum of London: www.museumoflondon.org.uk
The National Archives: www.nationalarchives.gov.uk
The Proceedings of the Old Bailey, London's Central Criminal Court, 1674 to 1913:
  www.oldbaileyonline.org
Oxford Dictionary of National Biography: www.oxforddnb.com
Princeton University: www.princeton.edu
UCL: www.ucl.ac.uk
UCLA Department of Epidemiology, School of Public Health, John Snow: www.ph.
  ucla.edu/epi/snow.html
UK Parliament: www.parliament.uk
UK Legislation 1267- Present: www.legislation.gov.uk
World Health Organization: www.who.int/topics/cholera/treatment/en
The Workhouse, The story of an instituition: www.workhouses.org.uk

**LECTURES**
Dr Bonnie Bassler, How Bacteria "Talk": http://ed.ted.com/lessons/how-bacteria-talk-
  bonnie-bassler
Dr Rita Colwell, *Climate Change, Oceans and Infectious Disease: Cholera Pandemics
  as a Model*, Annual Conference of the Society of General Microbiology, April 2014,
  www.youtube.com/watch?v=KvBuDxwV11Y

# Index

Broad Street/Broad Street Pump, 13, 129 – 161, 203 See also *Broadwick Street*

Broadwick Street, 8, 140 See also *Broad Street*

Brown, Dr Joseph, 37, 145

Budd, Dr William (1811-1880), 12 - 14, 50, 65, 129, 154 - 158, 179, 181, 186

Calcutta, 17, 174, 191 See also *Bay of Bengal, India, Jessore, River Ganges*

Calomel (Mercurous Chloride), 30, 31, 43

Canals, 13, 22, 50, 51, 52, 53, 55, 63, 183, 187, 202 See also *Aquatic Environment, Canals, Estuaries, Rivers, Waterways*

Carden, George Frederick (1798 – 1874), 113

Chadwick, Edwin (1800 – 1890), 66, 67, 69 - 71, 73 - 78, 85, 86, 96, 102. 103, 106, 123, 124, 125, 129, 154

Cholera,

Asiatic, 13, 15, 16, 34, 37, 38, 43, 45, 82, 104, 105, 140, 149, 174, 176

Bacterium, 17, 21, 22, 24, 25, 27, 28, 51, 62, 191, 195, 201, 202-3

Bill See *Nuisances Removal Acts*

Endemic, 201, 203

English, 16, 26, 43, 176

Epidemic, 27, 43, 62, 100, 107, 112, 191, 196, 201

Morbus, 15, 16, 18, 22, 32, 34

Prevention Act, 53, 57, 118

Spasmodic, 15, 117

See also Vibrio cholerae

Civil Registration Acts, 58, 101 - 104, 112

Clanny, Dr William Reid (1776 – 1850), 38 - 41, 44

Clemens, Professor Dr John, 192

Climate, 9, 10, 17, 19, 38

Coatbridge, 51 – 52

Colwell, Dr Rita R., 13, 200 – 203

Cooper, Edmund (1818 – 1893), 145, 152

Corn Laws, 70

Cresy, Edward (1792 – 1858), 68

Crohn's disease, 23 - 24, 136America, 11, 18, 69, 73, 100, 129, 130, 195, 200

Crossness, 167, 169, 189, 190

Cubitt, William (1785 – 1861), 69

Curtis, Dr Val, 63

Cyanobacteria, 23

Davies, Dr David (c.1822 – 1894), 179, 181, 186

Dhaka, Bangladesh, 27

Diarrhoea/Diarrhoeal Disease, 15, 28, 29, 39, 63, 82, 108, 109, 140, 141, 148, 149, 176, 177, 178, 181, 185, 189

Dickens, Charles (1812 – 1870), 68, 79, 93, 94

Diptheria, 15

Disease Maps 22, 145 – 146, 197

Disraeli, Benjamin (1804 – 1881), 166

Dougan, Professor Gordon, 7, 195,

DOVE (Delivering Oral Vaccine Effectively), 192, 193

Drainage, drains, 14, 42, 47, 53, 57, 60, 64 - 68, 76, 83, 85, 149, 151 - 153, 160, 162, 164 - 166, 175, 180, 183, 187, 189

INDEX

# INDEX

Sack, Professor David A., 7, 193

Salinity, 26, 27, 200

Sanitary Acts, 65, 186

Sanitation, 14, 19, 22, 56, 60, 63, 65, 67, 75, 76, 78, 91, 112, 132, 137, 154, 158, 163, 164, 170, 175, 181, 186,187, 193, 197, 199

Scarlatina, 37

Sedgwick, William T. (1855 – 1921), 129, 146

Senior, Nassau (1790 – 1864), 70, 73, 96

Serogroups, 26, 27, 194

Sewell, Dr John, 47

Shapter, Dr Thomas (1809 – 1902), 56, 57, 104, 118 – 121

Sheerness, 56, 188

Shoreditch, 181, 185,

Simon, Dr John (1816 – 1904), 78, 107, 129, 158, 159, 160, 161, 175, 176, 185, 186

Simpson, James (1799 – 1869), 138, 165, 179

Smallpox, 15, 21, 25

Snow, Dr John (1813 – 1858), 8, 13, 22, 24, 58, 82, 111, 125, 129, 130 – 146, 149, 151, 153 – 163, 169, 176, 178, 179, 185, 194, 196, 197, 203

Society for the Abolition of Burials in the Cities and Towns, 123, 126

Soho, 8, 129 - 161, 162, 203

Southampton, 125, 174 – 179

Southwark, 56, 63, 95, 105, 125, 135, 136, 138, 162, 169, 188

Southwark and Vauxhall Water Company, 125, 138, 139, 159 – 161

Southwood Smith, Dr Thomas

(1788 – 1861), 66, 67, 73, 75, 76, 77, 78, 85, 86

Speenhamland System, 70

Sproat, William, 39, 41

Stangate Creek, 34, 56

Stephenson, Robert (1803 – 1859), 68, 69, 131

Stepney, 56, 75, 182, 185

Sunderland, 22, 37, 38, 39, 40 - 46, 50, 51, 55, 56, 180

Swayne, Dr Joseph Griffith (1819 – 1903), 156, 158, 163

Sydenham, Thomas (1624 – 1689), 16, 26

Syphilis, 21

Teddington Lock, 137, 183

Temperance, intemperance, 43, 44, 54, 58

Temperance Movement, 133

Thomson, Professor Nicholas, 7, 193 – 194

*Times, The*, 12, 23, 31, 40, 43, 45 - 48, 56, 58, 67, 80, 88, 108, 127, 160, 162, 164, 166, 174, 176, 180, 181, 186, 189

Trade, Board of, 183

Trade/Trade Routes, 11, 12, 17, 22, 42, 43, 51, 69, 73, 131, 170

Trades Unions, 60, 70, 173

Tuberculosis, 15, 61

Tweedie, Dr Alexander, 37

Typhoid Fever, 12, 15, 156, 179, 187

Typhus, 21, 32, 75, 94

University College London, 102, 134

Hospital, 89

Utilitarianism, 73 – 74

Vaccines, 15, 191 – 193